Living through Cancer: Memoirs of a Canvivor

Revised Edition

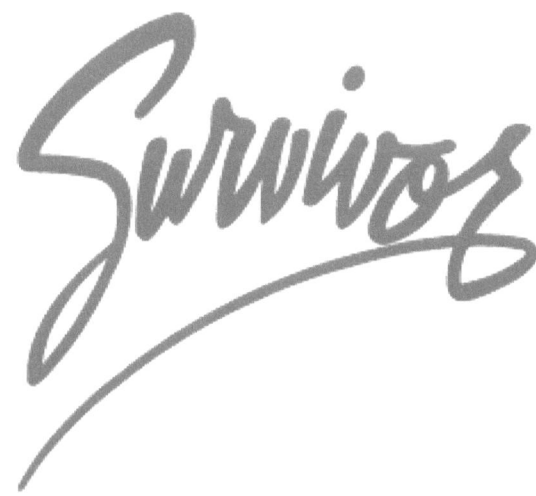

Felix Paul

January 2020

Living through Cancer: Memoirs of a Canvivor

Dedicated to:

The memory of my mother whose spirit has been my guardian angel, protecting and guiding me all along, more so since I was diagnosed with cancer in January 2008;

My wife who has been a pillar of strength all through my cancer journey, nourishing my body, mind, and spirit and inspiring hope that my cancer can be put behind;

Our children and their families who have stood by us all the while, loving, encouraging and supporting us in every possible way;

My medical team, past and present, to whom I owe my recovery and well-being in large measure;

Cancer patients and cancer survivors the world over with whom I share a bond.

Table of Contents

Acknowledgements

I would like to thank all those who made it possible for me to bring out this book. Among others, there are those who encouraged me to share my story with others, devoted time for a discussion of its content and design, offered comments and suggestions and helped improve its readability. I owe them all a great deal.

A special word of thanks to Thomas, my son-in-law, for formatting this revised version of the book.

Preface

"You hear the word 'cancer', and you think it is a death sentence" - Clare Balding

What is so scary about cancer? Almost everything! If you have cancer, you feel like being in a physical and emotional mess. You lose your appetite gradually, get weaker day by day, isolate yourself from others, become increasingly indifferent to your routine, and sink into a lassitude never experienced before. Cancer may also demoralize you to such an extent that you do not feel like yourself anymore; it seems like you have now been transformed into a weakling incapable of looking life in its face and meeting its multifarious challenges.

But why do you dread cancer much more than any other disease? It is largely because you know but too well that there is no known cure for cancer, despite what your doctors may suggest by way of treatment. You begin to harbour hitherto unknown fears that your life may come to a grinding halt any time soon; that you may lose your livelihood and find yourself in difficult personal circumstances; that the treatments your doctors suggest may rob you of your hard-earned money and force you to borrow heavily; that cancer being what it is, may reappear anytime and any number of times, though your doctors may say you are now cancer-free. It is as though you had been hit by lightning, or some evil power had cast a spell on you with a dark and sinister design.

Your fears may also be due to your awareness that conventional cancer treatment options are limited, as summed up aptly in the title of the cancer documentary, *Cut Poison Burn* (1). The only three treatment options available at present are surgery, chemotherapy and radiation therapy. There is no guarantee, however, that these much-touted treatments will bring about a long-lasting remission, let alone a permanent cure. Besides, there is always the risk of the treatments aggravating your condition and killing you even faster. It is small wonder, therefore, that many cancer patients, largely those who cannot afford the treatment costs, often turn to quacks who have little or no idea of cancer or its treatment methods. And you know with what results!

But is the cancer treatment scenario so dubious or unreliable as some may claim? Not necessarily. Surgery, chemotherapy and radiation therapy have for long been regarded as standard medical treatments for cancer. They may not always cure cancer, but there is no denying their usefulness in controlling the spread of disease and extending human life. However, if that is all these conventional therapies can achieve, it is awfully little. What seems to be sadly lacking in today's cancer care is the awareness that it may help to look for complementary or additional support from other systems of medicine. Alternative treatments embodying the core idea that many types of cancer can be prevented, controlled and even cured with a modified lifestyle are now gaining ground.

Studies show that a simple, stress-free life supported by a balanced diet, positive thinking, adequate sleep and regular physical exercise may go a long way in preventing and controlling cancer. Changing over to a healthy lifestyle would mean controlling risk factors that may trigger or aggravate cancer. In a sense, the secret of preventing or fighting cancer seems as simple as this: change over to a healthy lifestyle which will, in turn, augment your immunity levels and keep you healthy. Incidentally, there are well- documented stories of cancer patients who have modified their lifestyles and stayed cancer-free all their life.

My tryst with cancer

I was first diagnosed with cancer in 2008. Like most others, I went through surgery and six cycles of chemotherapy after which my doctors said I was *completely cured.* But the disease erupted again in 2011, and the earlier treatments, namely surgery and chemotherapy, were repeated with greater intensity. Hardly seven months later there was yet another recurrence; this time around, the issue was an infected lymph node in the abdominal area, which turned out to be the worst that could ever happen to me.

The oncologist explained that the cancer had metastasized, meaning that it had now turned footloose and travelled to a distant location. In all likelihood, it would turn more aggressive and spread to other parts of the body sooner rather than later. It seemed there was no way my life could be saved, except by repeating the earlier treatments supplemented by radiation therapy and targeted chemotherapy.

As suggested by my medical team, I had the infected lymph node removed surgically and went ahead with radiation therapy. At the end of it all, I was so devastated in body, mind and spirit that I began to wonder if my body could tolerate any further treatment. An inner voice kept warning me of an impending disaster if I were to go ahead with conventional treatments any further. Taking courage into my hands and well-supported by my family, I explored the possibility of switching to some alternative therapy as a last resort. Among the options considered, naturopathy (2) seemed profoundly significant in view of its core philosophy that physiological malfunctions of any kind can be corrected with a modified lifestyle.

Infused with fresh hopes that I could still beat the odds, I decided to try the new line of treatment for what it was worth. For me, it all began as an experiment but it turned out to be a well-established routine a little later. And the outcome, over the years, has been remarkable. It has now been about twelve years since I was first diagnosed and eight years since I changed over to the new lifestyle. I am still cancer-free. I eat and sleep well, exercise regularly, enjoy travelling and visiting people and, in short, live as active a life as in my pre-cancer days. And I hope to be able to go on cancer-free as long as I live.

About this book

The objective of this book is to share with you the lessons I have learned during my cancer journey of about twelve years. Cancer struck me at a point of time when I thought I was hale and healthy, and the diagnosis shocked me beyond words. The physical and emotional side effects of the treatments that followed were truly debilitating, and there were times during my cancer journey when I felt like crying out loud as Job did: "I loathe my life, I do not want to go on living"(3).

I would have easily given up and succumbed to my distressing circumstances had it not been for the mercy of God as manifested through the love, care and support I received from my wife, our children and their families. I am beholden in no small measure to the abiding care of my medical team as well as the wishes, greetings and prayers of relatives and friends. I feel grateful that I have arrived this far in my cancer journey, and I hope that my current state of remission will continue leading to a permanent cure.

My message through this book is this: Never ever give up hope whatever your stage of cancer. If you are a believer, have faith in your God that he is there to work it out for you. Trust your medical team and all others who love and care for you. Most of all, take responsibility for your well-being, as it is your life at stake, and as you need to care for it more than anyone else. Try and be positive in your approach and brave and relentless in your battle with cancer. With right decisions made, with right attitudes and with determination to fight and win, you can navigate successfully and emerge cancer-free one fine morning.

Why Canvivor?

Why do I call myself a canvivor – a word that no dictionary of English includes – instead of the familiar 'cancer survivor'? I thought I needed a more inclusive, a more telling term that would imply much more than 'someone with cancer who is still living'. I wanted to assume a name typical of someone in remission – someone with a tenuous, disruptive psyche that keeps them in a perpetual state of uncertainty about their health. Even false symptoms may throw them off their balance and make them wonder if their cancer is back. The bottom line is that being in remission is not as enviable as many may think; it may, on the contrary, be psychologically taxing and emotionally draining. It is on this account that I found 'cancer survivor' inadequate, which I replaced with 'canvivor' – a term I coined to convey my own meaning. For me 'canvivor' is as truly representative of my tenuous emotional state as of my disease-and-treatment-ravaged body and I am happy with the word.

Before you begin reading

I think a note of caution would be in order before you begin reading my story. The ideas, views and opinions expressed in this book are my own, and on no account do I want to thrust them on you. You may try any or all of what worked for me and the outcome may be as good as it was for me, if not better. But don't feel bad or discouraged, if the results you get at the end of the day are not as good as you expected. There could be any number of reasons why this is so, and this is no place to go into the details. My suggestions may therefore supplement and not necessarily replace what your doctor has suggested for you.

I wish you good luck!

Chapter 1: Life interrupted

"Now it is cancer's turn to be the disease that doesn't knock before it enters" –Susan Sontag, Illness as Metaphor

Episode 1

The physician looked up after viewing my blood test report. "This has come out pretty clean. You're borderline hypertensive. Your total cholesterol level may not be perfect, but it's well within the low-risk range. Everything else is fine," he said.

He looked into my eyes enquiringly for a while and added, "I'll prescribe some drugs, and we'll review your case after six months. Any questions?"

Obviously, he had nothing more to say and 'any questions?' was just a reminder that it was time for me to leave, and let the next patient come in. There was a small crowd of 'master-health-checkup' people waiting outside the physician's cubicle, and he had to see them all before 5 pm. Like his patients, the physician was in a hurry to finish this routine and turn to other things.

"Any questions?" This kept ringing in my ears for a few seconds, and I was wondering what to say. As a matter of fact, my lifestyle had been good, and so had been my medical history. To my knowledge, I had experienced no serious health issue of any kind, any time in the past. Now that I was expected to raise something, let me tell him

about a very minor thing that had of late been annoying –
persistent constipation. I just mentioned it for what it was
worth.

"How long have you had this?"

"For about six months now."

"How often do you have bowel movements?"

"Three or four times a week."

"What's the stool like?"

"At times it's dry and stone-like and difficult to pass."

"Do you have constipation and diarrhoea
alternately?"

"No, only constipation."

"Are you being treated for the condition now?"

"Not really. But when it gets intolerable, I take
antacids and laxatives."

"Any improvement?"

"Yes and no. There is some relief, but, by and large,
the problem still persists."

"Have you ever found anything odd about your
stool?"

Anything odd? I really did not understand. I was
wondering what to say when the physician came in again.

"Like blood, for instance?"

"Yes, rarely though. There is an occasional trace of blood."

"Have you done any bowel tests recently? Like colonoscopy (1) for instance?"

I thought I had heard the word before, but I hardly knew what the procedure would be like.

"No."

"Well, I suggest you do it now. You may see me again, if necessary."

The doctor rang up the hospital gastroenterologist for an appointment for me, wrote out a prescription, and said, "You can see the gastroenterologist now to schedule your colonoscopy. As I said, it's time you did it."

৯ ৯ ৯

It was early January 2008. The Coimbatore hospital where I had my master- health-checkup was a private healthcare centre with ambitious plans to expand and acquire a super-specialty status. Situated on a sparse piece of land along one of the arterial roads of the city, it largely catered to the middle-class with reasonably qualified and hardworking medical professionals on its staff.

The gastroenterologist to whom I carried a referral was a middle-aged man with a benign look. He viewed the report, raised his head, smiled and said,

"When do you want to do this?"

"Maybe tomorrow?"

"Not tomorrow. How about next week, next Wednesday to be precise?"

I nodded in agreement.

Asking me to lie down, he examined my tummy, pressing and tapping on the abdomen. He said he saw no reason anything could be wrong with me, but the colonoscopy would tell more.

He smiled again and said, "So, we'll meet again next Wednesday".

The doctor's assistant gave me a sheet of paper asking me to fill in certain details. She told me how to prepare for the colonoscopy.

"The day before the procedure, stop eating solids by 12 noon. You may then have clear liquids like fruit juice or black tea, but even this should stop by seven in the evening."

She pointed at the doctor's prescription slip and said,

"Get these drugs at the hospital pharmacy before you go home. And this is what you need to do by way of preparation," she said, putting into my hands, a printed sheet of instructions.

"Follow this step by step. Avoid eating or drinking anything on the morning of the procedure. I'd like you to report here on Wednesday by 8 am."

As my wife and I returned home, it was late in the evening, and we were completely fagged out. Living abroad, we had just landed in India on a short visit. The trip was intended to be a holiday, and we were looking forward to a good time with family and friends. We had packed quite a few items into our holiday agenda like travelling and meeting people some of whom we had not seen for years. The most significant item on the agenda was, however, my deceased father's birth centenary.

We had planned a small celebration in Thanjavur where my father is laid to rest in the cemetery adjacent to the cathedral. On the morning of the centenary day, there was to be a thanksgiving mass in the cathedral followed by a family get-together. Invitations had already been sent out to relatives and friends, and we were looking forward to a happy time.

Viewed in this context, the colonoscopy scheduled for the following week seemed a time-waster that had unexpectedly got in the way. It was upsetting to think that we had to wait for a week doing nothing until the procedure got over. This new development made it necessary to reschedule our programme by deleting a few items from our agenda.

"I wonder", I said," if I can skip the procedure for now. It's my gut feeling that my health is in good shape as it has always been, so nothing alarming may show up in the test. It would just be a waste of precious time and money."

"Penny-wise, pound-foolish," said my wife. "God forbid, but what if the test reveals something?"

"Something serious? You seem to think rather negatively and I wonder why".

"Look", said my wife, a little impatiently.

"You're already into your sixties, and, at this stage of life, you can't take health for granted. Did you say, it's a waste of time? How stupid! It's all fine if the outcome is as desired, but what if it happens to be otherwise? Either way, it's a win-win situation for you."

I was not pleased with what she said, and she understood as much.

"I know there won't be anything wrong," she said, trying to placate me." It's just that you shouldn't take chances where health is concerned. It's not for nothing that your doctor has suggested the test and to skip it wouldn't be wise."

I knew that, as a rule, my wife had the last word on matters of a serious nature, and she had almost always been right. Besides, the hospital visit had been so exhausting that I was in no mood to argue. It was time to go to bed which we did after praying for family and friends.

Episode 2

The gastroenterologist stopped the procedure midway, raised his eyes and looked at his assistant. The images he saw on the computer monitor set him thinking.

"Do you see the mass just above the sigmoid colon (1)? What do we make of it?" he said.

His assistant, a medical intern, was possibly a novice in interpreting medical scans. He nodded rather reluctantly as though he was not that sure.

"There's a stricture over there obstructing the scope. It could well be a tumour," the gastroenterologist said.

Still unsure, the assistant peered into the image and said,

"Yes, it looks like one."

Listening to their dialogue, I was alerted to a fresh concern that hit me like a bolt from the blue. I was then lying on my left side as the colonoscopy was in progress and feeling a little woozy from the sedation given earlier. Well within my viewing distance was the computer monitor that kept flashing image after image of the mazy folds of the insides of my colon. At first, the images were all pink and healthy-looking, but the scope stopped at a point where the image was very different - dark and sinister-looking.

It was this image on the monitor that the two medical professionals were so concerned about. The gastroenterologist took one more look at it and gestured to the nurse that there was nothing more to do. It took me some time to understand that the procedure had ended abruptly in about fifteen minutes. Didn't the doctor say it would take around forty-five minutes?

I started to experience something of a panic attack. Was anything the matter with me as my wife had suspected? My prophetic wife! I recalled the words she spoke the other day which seemed to reverberate through the procedure room, even as an uneasy sensation began to take hold of me. Anxious to know what was happening, I looked in the direction of the doctor who had now moved to a corner of the room. Between them, the doctor and his assistant were having a word in private. The lights were on again, and the nurse helped me get up.

"The procedure is over. The doctor is at his desk waiting to talk to you," she said.

Anxious to know what was coming on, I moved towards the doctor's desk with vague apprehensions. The doctor smiled as usual, though, it seemed, it was more in sympathy this time.

"Not very good news, I'm afraid," he said rather apologetically.

"What I could do for you was a sigmoidoscopy (2),

not a full colonoscopy as we had planned earlier. The scope would not proceed beyond a point, possibly because of some obstruction just above the sigmoid colon. There's nothing certain however that can be read from this," he said as though trying to calm my mind.

He went on. "A CT scan would tell us more. It produces images that highlight the problem, if any, and how widespread it is. Besides, the scan would clarify beyond doubt whether surgery is going to be helpful."

A little later, I found myself in the radiology wing of the hospital. A junior nurse made me do a few preliminaries for the oncoming scan. She started an IV on me and, inserting the needle of a loaded syringe into the IV tube, injected the medicine. Already tired, I began to drift off.

"Paul," shouted the radiologist's assistant, shaking off my daze and involuntarily putting me on my feet. Never before had I heard my name screamed out at such a volume. Well, I knew it was my turn to get in.

"Take off your clothes and wear this," the assistant said, handing me what looked like a bedroom gown. I moved into the radiology room where the radiologist greeted me with a grim smile.

"It's a simple procedure. It'll be over in 30 minutes," he said.

The procedure was short and simple and did not take longer than the radiologist had predicted. I looked at the radiologist for some clue on what he had found, but he was tight-lipped.

"You may return to the gastroenterologist now. He'll tell you everything you need to know," he said in a deep, ominous, baritone voice.

The wait at the gastroenterologist's room was long and agonizing. An hour and a half had passed before I was called in.

"Do you see this?" said the doctor, pointing to an image on the computer monitor that made little sense to me.

"As I guessed, it's a tumour that needs to be removed surgically. Not sure if it's benign or malignant, though," he said, as though to put me at ease. Strangely, he was not smiling this time.

The gastroenterologist went on to explain:

"Benign tumours are not cancer. They can be surgically removed and usually do not come back. More importantly, they do not spread to other parts of the body. As different from this, malignant tumours are cancer. Cancer cells can infiltrate into tissues and, much worse, can invade organs."

"The good news is your condition is treatable. Fortunately, the abnormality is confined to a part of the colon, and the right thing to do just now is to have it removed."

I had stopped listening to the doctor. Too dazed to comprehend anything! Whatever he was saying only fell on deaf ears. The only word I could hear was 'cancer' which kept echoing in my mind, horrifying me and chilling me to the bone.

How miserable! Too many visits to specialists and too much trouble! It was all like a vicious circle of visits around the entire hospital, first to the physician, followed by further visits to the gastroenterologist and the radiologist. And now I was at the surgeon's door. So, what next?

Unaware of what was passing through my mind, the gastroenterologist was still staring at me blankly, as we thanked him and got up to leave.

Chapter 2: Bracing for the storm

"You never know how strong you are until being strong is the only choice you have" - Cayla Mills

Episode 1

Back home from the hospital, I was apprehensive as the trauma of potential colorectal cancer (1) began to haunt me. True, I had not been diagnosed with cancer officially as yet. The gastroenterologist did not say it was cancer in so many words; neither did the diagnostic tests reveal anything conclusive. But I knew, in my heart of hearts, what I had been diagnosed with. The gastroenterologist knew it as well, but he would not formally confirm it before the pathology report (2) arrived. Apart from the doctor's studied reticence which spoke volumes, there was something strikingly different about his body language as he interpreted the test results – his quivery voice, unsteady eye contact and, of course, his characteristic smile that was conspicuously missing. All this conveyed a message that felt portentous.

Very bad news indeed! I was sitting speechless on the couch trying to think. Never before had I felt so dumb, so confused and so depressed. My mind was engulfed in a thick fog, and, however hard I tried, there seemed no way I could clear through it. Hazy and muddled scene after scene of what would happen in the days ahead hastened across my mind with every aspect of every scene feeling scary. Where was I headed? Would I be strong enough to confront my enemy head-on? Or would I have to admit defeat and meekly surrender to the oppressor? In addition to the physiological toll that surgery and other treatments would together exact of me, I would also have to journey through times that might be emotionally exhausting. Would I be able to cope with it all?

The first-ever issue to resolve was if I could go ahead with my job abroad. It seemed there was no way I could save my job if I decided to get treated in India. Second, would my wife and I be able to go through the ordeal of surgery and the follow-up on our own, or should we involve our children as well? Our daughter who lived in Coimbatore would willingly put herself out for us, and our son had already volunteered to be with us for as long as we would need his help. Together, they would help organize further medical tests, doctor appointments and hospital visits. Third, what would the treatment expenses be like? I had some hard-earned money put away in bank securities, but cancer treatment costs being what they were said to be, my savings seemed meagre. What would I do just in case I needed more money for my treatment? Besides, where would I have the treatment? In Coimbatore, Chennai or Mumbai?

The scariest part of it all was the question of my survival. I had read stories of people being diagnosed with cancer and succumbing to it in a matter of months. How long would I possibly live? Would the cancer diagnosis be the beginning of the end of my life's journey? Not that I was being pessimistic, but, no matter how hard my doctors tried to save my life, I might still die. Just in case - God forbid - I died while being operated on, or soon after the treatments, wouldn't my wife be devastated? Wouldn't she be left all alone? All our four children had their own families to look after, with on-going careers in front of them. No doubt, they would willingly look after and care for her, if she chose to live with them, but wouldn't it be hard on them to be with her in Coimbatore over a period of time? Wave after wave of scary thoughts rushed through my mind adding to my dismay.

I knew it for a fact that negativity of any kind would only aggravate my condition and might even kill me faster. What I needed in place of fear and anxiety was hope and confidence that I would ultimately triumph, no matter how long and hard the battle. Cultivating a positive attitude would eventually lead to a healthy mindset which in turn would promote physical health. If only I could shed my negativity and put in place a positive, healthy mindset! That would enable me to accept my situation as part of reality, help activate my inner strengths and inspire me to get down to brass tacks - the nitty-gritty of what needed to be done to put my health back on track- without further delay. But accepting the situation as part of reality! Therein lay the rub. It was easier said than done.

Brushing aside my ruminations for the moment, I

turned to my wife who was seated right in front of me. An expression of suppressed shock played over her face, but she was strangely quiet as though the turn of events that day had taken a toll on her ability to speak. How I wished she would break her silence and say something – maybe just a word that could inspire hope and confidence! Despite her apparent calm, I could see she was greatly troubled at heart. I could understand her feelings now as one who had lived with her for more than three decades. Disturbed as she was, it would be heartless to project my own emotion on her. I would let her remain so as long as she wanted, or until I found it appropriate to engage her in a conversation.

My thoughts on the need for a positive mindset having returned, I began to wonder how I could accept my situation as part of reality. Was there any way I could come to terms with my enemy, any way I could relate to my cancer, any way I could identify with it? If I could, that would go a long way in mitigating my shock and suffering. But why in the first place did cancer pick me up from among so many for this singular visitation? I thought over the question long and hard, and it suddenly flashed across my mind that I *did* have a kinship of sorts with my cancer – it ran in my family. Strange that I had not thought of it earlier! As a matter of fact, I should never have been surprised at the diagnosis in the first instance! Cancer took my father when he was just forty years of age, and my eldest sister when she was fifty-four. And it was colorectal cancer in either case!

I was seven years old when my father died - too young to understand the intensity of his suffering. But I recalled my mother telling me and my siblings about the intensity of his suffering. He had for long been complaining of a pain in the abdomen but kept ignoring it until one day it turned excruciating. It was then that he was diagnosed with terminal stage colorectal cancer and there was nothing much his doctors could do to save his life. Equally painful and gruesome was my sister's battle with cancer. She had hardly turned fifty when she started having symptoms like weight loss, extreme fatigue, abdominal cramps and loss of appetite. She had been treated for these symptoms now and then, but no one ever guessed it could be anything serious. Spiritual and stoic as she had always been, she accepted her suffering as divine will. By the time she was diagnosed, her condition had turned metastatic, and her last days were miserable.

Given this family history, how come it never occurred to me that I could be the next cancer victim in my family line? By mid-2007, I had lost considerable weight, and everyone attributed it to my mother's death in December 2006. I believed it myself because her death was a personal loss to me, and it took me quite some time to recover from the shock. Besides, I began to experience symptoms like loss of appetite and sleep deprivation which, I thought, were due to my advancing age. And I was also getting irritable more and more - even trifles putting me off and making me fly into a rage. But the most pronounced symptom was my frequent bouts of constipation which would sometimes persist for days together. Strangely, the thought never crossed my mind that all this could be symptomatic of something serious.

Well, I had my kinship with cancer clearly defined now. Cancer needed someone for a victim in my generation, and it just happened to be me. Viewing my cancer dispassionately, I could not miss its *partiality* to me. For one thing, it had delayed striking me until I was well into my sixties, and the physical and emotional suffering I underwent subsequently was possibly far more tolerable than what my father or my sister would have experienced. It hit me at a stage when I was rather complacent about my life in general; my life had been good and my career even better taking me to heights I had never imagined I would ever be able to reach. Besides, my children had all been married and well-settled in life, so there was nothing more that I could desire. There was, of course, my wife to think of, but I knew she would not be left behind needy or insecure, and my children would be supportive just in case she needed anything more.

At the end of this enlightenment, it was no longer that difficult for me to accept my situation as part of reality. From then on, questions of a self-pitying nature such as "Why me?" or "What have I done to deserve this? would not bother me anymore. One could keep asking such questions endlessly, but I knew there were no answers. For one thing, no one - good or bad, young or old, rich or poor - deserves this disease. Cancer, like death, is a leveller that lays its icy hand on whomsoever it pleases and brings them to dust. In a way, it is as inscrutable as the Almighty himself, what with its quirky whimsicalities, unpredictable visitations, weird modes of affliction and mysterious patterns of remissions and recurrences. You either face it squarely or succumb to it meekly. As for me, I would not just face it, but take it by its horns for whatever the fight was worth.

Episode 2

Vowing to fight is not synonymous with winning; it is just an essential first step towards winning. To be able to fight and win, I needed to empower myself, in the first instance, with as much information about the enemy as I possibly could. No doubt, what was known of cancer at that point of time was very little, but most of it all was scientifically verified and well-documented. Getting to know my enemy inside out would help me join forces with my medical team so that informed decisions on treatment options could be taken. It would enable me, in particular, to stay focused on my onerous mission – confronting and fighting an enemy who threatened to take my life. I set about acquiring as much information on cancer and cancer treatments as I could, from a variety of sources including websites, books, journals and newspaper articles.

What is cancer?

Cancer is the Latin translation of the Greek word,

karkinos, which means 'crab'. Hippocrates (460-370 BC), the Father of Medicine, was the first-ever to use the crab analogy to describe the disease, possibly because he had noticed that the swollen veins around a malignant tumour resembled the limbs of a crab. The history of cancer shows that from time immemorial human beings, as well as animals, have been afflicted with different kinds of cancer. It is said that there are about two hundred different types of cancer (1), each with its own distinguishing characteristics. All the same, cancers share some characteristics in common, the most typical of them being their ability to continue to divide and multiply perpetually.

In a healthy body, cells grow, divide into new cells and die in an orderly, time-bound way. This systematic process turns topsy-turvy when cancer strikes. Cells begin to multiply unchecked, and they do not die as normal cells do. This abnormal growth of cells leads to the formation of some swelling or lump which is generally referred to as a tumour. Left undetected, these malignant cells begin to spread to nearby tissues, and may even invade distant parts or organs of the body. When cancer spreads from its original location to distant body tissues or organs, the progression is called *metastasis.*

What causes cancer?

What causes cancer is still a mystery. Studies reveal that people with certain risk factors are more cancer-prone than others. Different cancers are said to have different risk factors. For example, being exposed to intense sunlight is a risk factor for skin cancer. Smoking is a risk factor for several cancers including cancers of the lungs, mouth, kidneys, bladder and colon. However, it does not necessarily mean that someone without any risk factor will *not* get cancer. It is equally false to assume that those who have one or more risk factors will necessarily get cancer. Further, even where a cancer patient is known to have one or more risk factors, it is hard to determine whether the person's cancer was triggered by those risk factors. No doubt, the risk-factor theory still remains a little vague where cancer is concerned, but the best procedure seems to be to steer clear of those risk factors that are said to cause a particular type of cancer.

What is colorectal cancer?

Colorectal cancer starts in the colon or the rectum. There are many types of cancers that start in some part of the colon, but most colorectal cancers are of a type called *adenocarcinomas* (2). As a rule, a colorectal cancer develops from a polyp or a growth on the inner lining of the colon or the rectum. A polyp can be benign or non-cancerous. Or it may be malignant or cancerous. A malignant polyp often grows into a cancerous tumour over a period of time. Cancer cells from the tumour eventually begin to grow into the wall of the colon or the rectum. When they spread outside the colon, they often invade the nearby lymph nodes. From there, they may travel further, and even reach distant organs such as the liver and the lungs.

Do lifestyle factors cause colorectal cancer?

Studies show that there is a strong correlation between colorectal cancer and lifestyle factors such as diet, body weight and exercise. As a rule, diets rich in fat and low in calcium and fibre may increase the risk of the disease. It is good to avoid red meats which are known to have a link with causing the disease. Cooking meats at very high temperatures is not desirable either, as it produces certain chemicals that may add to the risk of colorectal cancer. It is equally well-known that a diet rich in vegetables, fruits and whole grains can help minimize or reduce one's chances of getting the disease. Physical inactivity, smoking, alcohol abuse and obesity are additional factors that may cause colorectal cancer. It is also known that people with a family history of colorectal cancer have a greater risk of cancer - almost one in every five people with colorectal cancer has a family history of the disease.

What is staging? What do different colorectal cancer stages mean?

Staging refers to the extent to which disease has spread. Colorectal cancer has the following stages:

Stage 0: Cancer is found only in the innermost lining

of the colon or rectum.

Stage 1: Cancer has grown into the inner wall of the colon or the rectum but has not grown through the wall.

Stage 2: Cancer has grown through the wall invading nearby tissues but has not spread to the lymph nodes.

Stage 3: Cancer has spread to the lymph nodes, but not to any other part of the body.

Stage 4: Cancer has spread to other parts of the body as well, such as the liver or the lungs.

What treatment options are there for colorectal cancer?

To treat colorectal cancer, one or more conventional treatment methods such as surgery, chemotherapy or radiation therapy can be used. The oncologist decides which of the treatments comes first, depending on the location and staging of the disease. More often than not, surgery comes in first. The surgeon may remove only the diseased part of the colon, leaving the rest of the colon intact, but in rare cases, he may even decide to remove the entire colon. Once the surgery is done, adjuvant chemotherapy (3) may be administered either intravenously or orally. The chemotherapy administered may be a single drug or a combination of two or more drugs. Or the oncologist may administer one drug now, followed by one or more drugs later. In addition, radiation therapy may also be recommended to destroy or shrink a tumour, or to destroy cancer cells left behind after surgery.

Do cancer treatments have side effects?

Each of these treatments has its own share of side effects. Surgery is invasive, and it may leave behind not just a scar but some permanent physical disability. Chemotherapy may cause more suffering than even cancer. The range of side effects it may cause varies in intensity from a lowered appetite, nausea or diarrhea, to more serious, long-time or even permanent conditions such as a 'chemo brain' (characterized by muddled thinking, forgetfulness and inability to concentrate), and 'peripheral neuropathy' (damage to nerves leading to partial numbness in one's hands and feet). Radiation therapy may result in temporary conditions such as vomiting, diarrhoea and bloody stools, and may even lead to permanent conditions such as organ damage, incontinence and erectile dysfunction.

What are cancer treatment costs like?

It is a well-known fact that conventional cancer treatment costs have been escalating over the years. According to an estimate, costs including prices of drugs, doctor fees and hospital charges have risen by about seventy-five per cent in the last couple of decades. The American Cancer Society notes that in the U.S., though private insurance would take care of many of the costs of treatment, a patient's out-ofpocket costs might exceed one billion dollars per year. According to the American Institute of Cancer Research (AICR) (4), cancer treatment has always been more expensive than the treatment of any other disease. And it is getting more and more unaffordable, especially for patients without an insurance cover. It is said that if this situation goes on unchecked, cancer patients will eventually be forced to choose between successful and expensive treatments on the one hand and less effective and cheaper treatments on the other. Predictably, the outcome would be disastrous.

What are complementary and alternative medicines (CAM)?

I also gathered information on what is known as 'complementary and alternative medicines' (CAM). 'Complementary medicine' includes therapies that supplement or add to standard treatments such as surgery, chemotherapy and radiation therapy. 'Alternative medicine', as different from this, is a set of therapies that replace standard treatments. There is also another approach to cancer treatment called 'integrative medicine' which claims to be a 'whole-person' treatment inasmuch as it claims to care not merely for the patient's body, but his mind, and spirit as well. As a rule, these therapies are non-invasive and less expensive for the most part. Each of these therapies has its own powerful exponents who claim very positive results, though more than ninety per cent of cancer patients all over the world still prefer to get treated with conventional methods. One reason why this is so is that claims of the 'cures' attributed to some of these alternative therapies are largely anecdotal; they are not evidence-based or supported by authentic documentation.

Most importantly, my little research convinced me that there was still hope for me to put my disease behind and get back to a normal life. The good news is that *not* all cancer patients die of cancer. Conventional treatments of cancer are, no doubt, very uncomfortable and even painful, but it is good to remember that the life-threatening, almost desperate situation caused by cancer devastation calls indeed for an equally aggressive and desperate remedy. The hard, painful and expensive treatment options available at the moment are but a small price cancer patients have to pay in order to save their lives. All cancers, whatever the stages, are treatable, as seen in the case of millions of cancer survivors all over the world, who live to share stories of how they defeated cancer. God willing, I told myself, I could very well be one of them; I would live long enough to tell my own story of cancer for the benefit of all cancer patients, past and present.

Episode 3

Among other things, my little research on cancer convinced me of the need to own responsibility for my treatment and eventual well-being. Ahead of me was a long road, and I had to move along taking significant decisions on my way. After all, it was *my* life at stake, and it made perfect sense that I take responsibility for it. Being responsible would mean, among other things, accepting my condition as it was and working with my medical team closely - understanding and evaluating their suggestions, and helping them take appropriate medical decisions. An essential precondition to making it all feasible would be to trust my doctors in the first place; I needed to firmly believe that they were well-intentioned and honest, that they knew what they were expected to do, and that their suggestions would eventually lead to my recovery.

The following day, accompanied by my wife, I set out for my first meeting with the surgeon. It was early morning, and we made it a point to be at his surgery before the place got crowded. As we were getting in, we found that the narrow corridor leading to the surgery was already crowded with patients and visitors. Fortunately, the surgeon arrived on time, and, luckily, we were called in first. Starting off with a few personal queries to me, the answers to which he wrote down on a notepad, he viewed my chart and the referral from the gastroenterologist. Asking me to lie down, he repeatedly pressed and thumped on the abdomen just above the sigmoid colon, and his adept touch seemed to tell him quite a good deal.

Pointing at the image on the computer monitor, the surgeon began to explain the procedure to remove the tumour. I interrupted him for a while with a question that had for long been pestering me:

"Is this surgery absolutely necessary?"

What a question to ask a surgeon! I could see a flash of surprise play across his face for a few seconds. His surprise quickly changed to sympathy, and he went on to explain:

> "I wish I could say 'no', but my answer is a clear 'yes'. In your case, surgery is an essential first step in our treatment protocol."

I was disappointed. There was yet another question, though I knew what the answer was going to be like:

> "Do you think it's cancer?"

> "It's too early to say anything for certain. We need to keep our fingers crossed until we see the pathology report."

> It was now the surgeon's turn to ask questions: "Do you have a family history of cancer?"

I told him about my father and my sister who fell victim to colorectal cancer.

Taking down what I said on his notepad, he turned to me and said:

> "You do have a family history of cancer, so your risk is even greater. However, as

> I said just now, it's too early to say anything."

> He went on: "Have you ever had a surgery done

before?"

"None," I said.

The surgeon proceeded to explain the two surgical options open – laparoscopy (1) and open surgery (2). A well-acknowledged laparoscopic surgeon, he elaborated on the virtues of laparoscopy. He pointed out that he would in all probability do a laparoscopy rather than an open surgery. Before deciding, he would, however, have a word with his colleague.

"In matters such as this," he said, "discussion helps".

He took a much longer look at the computer image this time and said:

"I'm afraid I may have to remove a part of your rectum as well, if necessary, I'll then have to follow it up with a colostomy (3)."

I hardly knew what he was talking about, and he explained:

"Colostomy is a surgical procedure to make an opening on the abdominal wall to allow stool to be collected into a bag. The opening is temporary in most cases and will be closed soon after the rectum heals from surgery."

The idea that, in addition to being cut, I might also be gifted with a stinky colostomy bag was too hard to digest. I must have looked upset and pathetic, so the surgeon thought it prudent to allay my fear.

> "I didn't say, I am going to do a colostomy. I only said, 'if necessary'."

The surgeon advised me to undergo surgery in a day or two, but I was for putting it put off by a week or two. This was because of the oncoming celebration at Thanjavur a couple of days later in memory of my deceased father. While I appreciated the surgeon's advice in view of the urgency of the situation, there was no way I could postpone the event. My life was important, no doubt, but equally important to me was this celebration - a small gesture from a loving son to honour the memory of his dead father.

The surgeon agreed to have the procedure postponed to the third week of January 2008. He suggested that we check in at the hospital on the afternoon of the day of surgery. To begin with, there would be a few tests and some paperwork to do, all of which might take a couple of hours. The surgery would begin late in the evening and might be completed in about three hours.

As we were leaving, the surgeon got up and shook my hand.

> "There's nothing to worry. If anything, surgery will only make your life better," he said, smiling.

My father's centenary celebration at Thanjavur was both

joyful and solemn. There was a high mass in the diocesan church with the church choir in full attendance. This was followed by a visit to the church cemetery where my parents lie buried in the same grave. Once out of the cemetery, we exchanged greetings with our relatives and friends. It was nice meeting them, some of whom we had not seen for years.

Not far away was the hotel where we got together soon after the church service. Older relatives spoke admiringly of my father, and how they were impressed by his qualities of the mind and heart. The occasion turned solemn when mention was made of his untimely death, especially of his last days of extreme anguish, pain and misery. Rather than the physical pain, one of them said, what really devastated my father was the concern that he was leaving behind a young wife and four hapless children who were too young to know what growing up fatherless would be like. "But the merciful Lord," the person went on, "listened to the dying man's prayer by taking as good care of the widow and her children as he could have ever wished."

None in the gathering except my wife and children knew anything about my diagnosis, and it was good we did not tell anyone. Information about my diagnosis and the impending surgery would have only brought in a flood of unwanted sympathy as well as queries too many and perhaps too inconvenient to answer. Not that we were reluctant to share the unhappy news, but this was not the right time for it. The news would only defeat the very purpose of the function by turning it upside down and shifting the focus away from my father. It would be unfortunate if this ever happened. No, not now!

I had for quite some time put away thoughts of my cancer and the impending surgery, but now, having been reminded of how my father died, my thoughts returned and haunted me as though with a vengeance. Would I have to deal with so much as my father did, and would my cancer time be as devastating? True, I had vowed to take the monster by its horns, and fight as hard as I could, but would I be equal to the task? Or had I overrated my own powers, and challenged an enemy too strong, too ruthless and too savage for me to overcome? And how long would the battle go on – for months, years or decades? And even if I was fortunate to emerge triumphant, at what expense would it all be - to my body, mind and spirit? Would the outcome be worth the struggle, and would life be still livable? I could only ask questions.

Chapter 3: On being an inpatient

"It may seem a strange principle to enunciate as the very first requirement in a hospital that it should do the sick no harm" – Florence Nightingale

Episode 1

We returned to Coimbatore to prepare for our hospital stay. In just a couple of days, I would undergo my first ever surgery and might have to stay in the hospital for about ten days, or until the surgeon suggested I could be discharged without any risk of infection. Our son had already arrived and would be with us for as long as we needed his presence. Together, our son and daughter would do everything needed to make our hospital stay more comfortable and less stressful. Our other two daughters had been told to put off their visit to a later date, preferably after my discharge from hospital. They would be kept informed meanwhile of every single happening of significance at our end. It was such a comfort to know that all the family would stay in close touch, with two of our children personally attending on us during our hospital stay.

On the day I was scheduled for surgery, we checked in at the hospital by midday. The surgery was to be done late in the evening, and, to begin with, certain preliminaries had to be completed. A nurse in uniform started an IV on me, tied an identity band around my wrist, and instructed me not to eat or drink after 7 pm. She got some papers signed by me and my wife and said that the surgeon would arrive soon.

The surgeon greeted me as he entered, and the very first thing he asked me was about our Thanjavur trip.

"So," he said, "you've returned twice blessed - by God and your dad."

"Thrice blessed," I said, smiling. "Maybe I forgot to tell you that my parents lie buried in the same grave."

"You'd need all their blessings and much more. Now, coming to business, your surgery is scheduled for 10.30 pm and may end in about three hours. By the way, your blood work results have just come in, and everything is normal including your CEA (1)."

"What's CEA?" I said. The surgeon went on to explain:

"It's a blood tumour marker for certain types of cancers including colorectal cancer. CEA levels are measured before and after surgery to evaluate the success of the surgery done and the patient's chances of recovery. "

"You just said that my CEA is normal. Doesn't that mean I don't have cancer?"

"We don't usually jump to a conclusion taking only the CEA level into account. The CEA test is reliable as a baseline indication, but no medical professional would ever confirm disease entirely on its basis."

"So, chances are the tumour is not malignant?"

The surgeon's body language seemed to convey the message that he was not for taking any more questions of the kind.

"As I said earlier, we still don't know if the tumour is benign or malignant. It could very well turn out to be benign at the end of the day, but we can't sit back and assume. Benign or malignant, the tumour should go, and that's why we're moving on to surgery now. "

"Before the surgery," the surgeon added, "a few medical preliminaries such as an X-ray and ECG need to be completed. My assistant will be here in a short while to take you for the tests."

He looked into my eyes, and rightly guessed what I was thinking.

"I know you'd like to ask if these tests are necessary. Yes, it's all part of our surgical protocol. We need to ensure that there is no disease elsewhere and that your cardio health is good enough to withstand the rigours of surgery. As I said, you'll get through the procedure without a hitch. I'll see you again tomorrow. Meanwhile, good luck!"

"Tomorrow? What does he mean?" I asked the surgeon's assistant who had just arrived.

"Well, he would, of course, be the doctor doing the surgery. But he may not be there when you regain consciousness."

The surgeon's assistant helped me do the X-ray and then took me to the cardiologist.

The cardiologist verified my personal information, asked a few questions about my lifestyle, and went ahead with the procedure. At the end of it, he wrote out a quick report and gave it to the surgeon's assistant.

"Did I pass the test?" I said, smiling.

Clearly, the cardiologist did not expect this question, and he looked amused.

"With distinction," he replied, with a twinkle in his eye.

⇛ ⇛ ⇛

The preliminaries being over, I was wheeled back to the hospital room where my wife and son were waiting. My wife had missed sleep for more than a couple of days, and she looked tired and careworn. On the table close to where she was sitting, there was the Holy Bible which had always been her refuge at times of stress. Getting close to me and taking my hand into hers, she said,

"The Lord is there to protect you from all evil. It's all going to work out well for you, and you'll come out disease-free and healthy."

It was reassuring to listen to her kind words, and I *did* believe that her words would come true. It was past nine in the evening, and the call from the surgeon might come anytime now.

A little later, two very young attendants came along and helped me shift to a transit bed on wheels. I lay motionless, as they rushed me along the narrow corridor in great haste as though it was an emergency situation. My wife and my son hastened after me, making passersby wonder why I was being rushed in such haste. As we were moving to the waiting area adjoining the operation theatre, the attendants slowed down a bit and I thought it was time to say good-bye to my family. Tears had welled up in my wife's eyes, and my son was looking stunned and speechless. As I was about to say something to them, the attendants whisked me away into the waiting area.

Left alone in semi-darkness, I began to wonder if the procedure would go off well and if I would emerge alive from the surgeon's table. I could not help feeling that my time of reckoning had arrived. Before very late, I wanted to look back on my life, repent my sins and seek the Lord's forgiveness and mercy. It was also time to thank God for his numerous blessings which, a sinner as I had always been, I hardly deserved. The short spiritual exercise soon filled me with a feeling of peace and serenity I had never experienced before - a peace that defied every description, a serenity that could only come from God.

It was time for the procedure to start, and I was shifted to the surgeon's table. The anaesthetist (2) checked my name on my wrist, smiled, and said,

"Mr Paul?"

I nodded, and he went on.

"You're married?"

I nodded again.

"Do you smoke or drink?"

"I don't smoke, but I take a drink or two occasionally."

"No harm," he said, with a soft chuckle. "As a matter of fact, I drink at weekends, though I tell my patients not to. Do you exercise regularly?"

"That's something I can't do without," I said a little proudly.

"Well, your lifestyle will go a long way in helping you recover fast. Now I'm going to administer the anaesthetic. You may feel it a little bit, but don't worry, you'll be off in a few minutes. Good luck!"

My eyelids turned heavy soon after, and I was drifting away into a state of unconsciousness.

Episode 2

Regaining consciousness, I found myself abandoned on a

trolley bed in the waiting area. How strange! Wasn't *it* done yet? Perhaps they were still waiting for the surgeon, and I began to wonder why he was taking so long. With just one soft light glowing overhead, the place was almost dark, and the ambience was gloomy and dismal. I was feeling a little drowsy, as the anaesthetic was still working. I sensed some discomfort in my abdomen which felt strangely moist and tender. And my hand stumbled on what felt like tubes that crisscrossed the entire abdominal area. It struck me just then. The blessed procedure had already ended! How stupid! What I thought to be the waiting room was indeed the recovery room where patients were left to recover soon after surgery. Thank goodness! What a relief to know I was alive!

Not much later, I heard muffled voices that seemed to come from nowhere. Pricking up my ears, I listened. Clearly, there were people around, so I peered into the dark to see who they were, and what they were up to. There were three young women, hospital attendants, who broke into conspiratorial whispers and muted giggles alternately. Obviously, they were unaware that I was awake and listening. I heard a few names mentioned repeatedly, and, going by the excitement these names evoked, I understood it was all spicy in-house gossip. The young women were simply having a good time, exchanging juicy tales. They had chosen the spot for privacy, and the place, semi-dark and desolate as it was, seemed well-suited for their purpose. I turned away from them and fell back to sleep soon after.

When I awoke the next morning, I found myself back in our hospital room. It was so nice to see my wife and children again after what felt like ages. It was depressing, however, to find myself tied down to my hospital bed. With an IV attached to my arm, an oxygen mask covering half my face, and a nasogastric tube dropping through my nose, I must have been a spectacle to watch. I had several other tubes running from and into my body, including a catheter (1) to drain urine and another to drain the fluid collected at the surgical site. On top of it all, I had a large vertical incision across my umbilicus with retention sutures, and the whole area felt raw, tender and painful.

It was miserable lying on my back all the time with nothing much to view except the ceiling above and the wall opposite. I once tried to turn sideways, but it hurt so badly that I would not venture it again. Besides, I was feeling inexplicably weak and thoroughly exhausted. My throat was dry, and I was feeling thirsty. The very thought of eating was loathsome, though I had not eaten for more than twenty hours. The discomfort from bloating was so terrible that I kept wondering if some surgical tool had been inadvertently left behind in my abdomen. I remembered being told earlier that the first few days after the surgery would be very demanding, so the only thing I was *officially* expected to do was rest in bed. How funny! I was expected to *rest* in such condition, for as long as a week, if not more.

I was reminded of the amazing story of Dr James Esdaille

(2), a Scottish surgeon serving in India, who performed about 400 major surgeries between 1843 and 1846 with great precision, using little more than simple hypnosis and the power of suggestion. His patients experienced no great pain, and, what was more, there were no deaths during the operations. How unfortunate, I thought, modern surgery caused so much pain, damage and distress despite the giant strides medical science and technology had taken over the years! It was a pity, I told myself, that Dr Esdaille's simple surgical procedure had been replaced by complicated and patient-unfriendly surgical practices.

A little reflection convinced me however that all the discomfort I was having was but a necessary part of convalescence leading to my eventual recovery. Instead of being disgruntled, I told myself, I should feel not just relieved, but happy. Things were certainly looking up for me! The surgery had gone off without complications, the tumour had been removed, and the cancer had hopefully been put behind. I was fortunate to have a medical team that was truly caring. More than all, my family was there to give me the much-needed emotional support. What more would I possibly need under those circumstances? In a few more days I would go back home to return to a normal life. God willing, I would even go back to work.

I looked through the window that had just been thrown open to let in sunshine and fresh air. Warm and comforting, the January sun seemed to beckon to me to bask in its glory. The cool and gentle breeze seemed to waft to me a fragrance that was at once refreshing and soothing. The pale-yellow flowers dancing merrily on treetops looked as though they were out to greet me with a get-well message. Sparrows on tree branches were chirping happily around as though to deliver Mother Nature's tidings that everything would work out well for me. Not far beyond, there was the arterial highway that throbbed with unusual life - vehicles, big and small, were speeding along, perhaps because they had a long way to go, and a great deal to do before the day ended.

My brief but happy distraction ended abruptly when the surgeon walked in to ask how I was feeling. He explained why he chose to do an open surgery instead of a laparoscopy. He checked me all over, read the hospital chart, and seemed satisfied with my progress.

> "The pleasant side of the news is that your cancer is gone. What's more, you haven't got a colostomy bag," he said, smiling.

> "The unpleasant part of it is that you may need chemotherapy (3) with or without radiation therapy (4). The oncologist (5) will visit you soon to discuss what is needed as a follow-up," he added.

℞ ℞ ℞

Around midday, a desolate cry for help from one of the rooms closeby pierced through the peaceful ambience of the special ward. It was a shrill female voice that came from one of the rooms nearby, and people were seen rushing to it. Before long, news began to spread that the young patient occupying the room was having symptoms of a cardiac arrest. The duty doctor promptly arrived on the scene, and, on his instructions, the patient was removed to the ICU, and then to the operation theatre. This unfortunate turn of events evoked at once great empathy and excitement. Inquisitive faces popped through half-open doors, anxious to know what was unfolding. Elderly women, who had hardly known each other before, congregated into a small group to exchange whatever they knew about the young man and his family. Careworn and weary-looking, they seemed to take comfort at the thought that their own lot was far better than that of the young wife who cried out for help.

The surgery having been done, the patient was brought back to his room late in the evening. More news came along that he was a forty-something software techie working for an MNC. He had constantly been under enormous pressure to meet deadlines, attend project discussions and submit reports. Of late, work pressure had multiplied for him, and he had to slog for long hours so as to be able to survive in his organization. At the end of the long day, he would often return home totally exhausted. But, a loving husband and a devoted father as he had always been, he still found time to be with his family before going to bed. This routine would not, however, go on for long, and, one day, he was so badly indisposed that he had to consult a cardiologist. It was then that he was diagnosed with a heart problem.

The cardiologist put him on a strict diet and a mild exercise regimen. Drugs to control his BP and cholesterol levels were prescribed, and he was advised to sleep longer. The young man followed the doctor's instructions meticulously, and it seemed as though it was just a matter of time before he completely recovered. But, as ill-luck would have it, he contracted a bacterial sinus infection a little later, and the local GP he consulted prescribed a popular antibiotic. Unfortunately, it did not strike the young man that he should tell the GP about the drugs he was taking for his heart problem. As ill-luck would have it, there was an unwanted drug interaction with the antibiotic causing a severe allergy and aggravating his heart condition. The cardiologist chided the young man for taking the antibiotic without consulting him, but nothing much could be done to undo the damage the drug had caused. It was in such critical condition that he was brought to this hospital for treatment.

The patient's young wife had accompanied him to the hospital and, as the report had it, she was devoted to his care. The couple had four children aged between eleven and three years, and in view of their parents being away from home, they were now being looked after by their grandmother. At weekends the children would visit their sick father in the hospital, and the family would have a good time together however short it was. The two elder children seemed to have an inkling of what was happening, but the younger ones were blissfully unaware of the severity of their father's condition. They kept lamenting how they missed him and urged him to return home as early as he could. When it was time for the children to depart, it would be a moment of emotion for the father; he would see them off with tears in his eyes.

A couple of days later, the inevitable happened. The young man's condition began to deteriorate rapidly. His BP went down, his pulse fell dramatically, and he became almost breathless. He was removed to the ICU where he was put on a respirator and given life-saving drugs. By the time the cardiologist came along to see him, the patient's health had further deteriorated. He had slipped into a coma. The cardiologist advised a scan to ascertain his condition, and the film showed fresh lesions in his heart. Further tests were carried out to determine the cause of the deterioration, but before the results came in, the patient suffered a stroke. It seemed there was nothing much left that could be done to save his life.

What followed was heartrending. There wailing from inside the hospital room turned pathetic as more and more visitors arrived on the scene. The young widow sat by her dead husband's body, silent and stupefied. Sorrow had devastated her so intensely that she could neither cry nor speak. It was depressing to see the children crying their heart out, and others taking turns to console them. My memory flew back to times when my father died, leaving behind a young wife and four very young children. I was reminded of the hard times, struggles and insecurities my dear mother had to face after the tragedy. From then on she ceased to live for herself and strove relentlessly to raise me and my siblings. Caring for her children turned out to be her only mission in life, and she did it so well and so cheerfully.

How I wished this young widow would face the hard times ahead as ably as my mother did and be as successful! I silently prayed for her and her children before going to sleep.

Episode 3

The day dawned with a kind of normality that carried no remnants of the previous day's tragedy. The paramedics who stood by the bereaved family sharing their emotion just a day before were now engrossed in their routine as though what had happened was a normal, day-to-day occurrence. Equally busy with their work were the cleaners and the ward boys, as the ward supervisor went around shouting orders at them. In the absence of fresh fodder to feed on, the gossip group had dispersed temporarily, renewing their dedication to the patients under their care. The canteen boy went around knocking on doors to see if the patients and their attendants had got up for their morning tea. When, a little later, doctors started streaming in with junior doctors and nurses dancing attendance on them, the patients were already up and about wondering what the day had in store for them.

The gastroenterologist who was the first to visit me that day brought with him the much-awaited biopsy report.

"The biopsy has come back positive," he said, looking at me, intently.

He seemed truly sorry for me, but I turned away to avoid his expression of sympathy. My face registered no emotion, as the news was not unexpected. Now, what I was more concerned about was what stage my cancer was, and what decision had been taken on the question of chemotherapy for me. I had survived my fear of death, but now it was this horror of chemotherapy. Out of the frying pan into the fire? What was it about chemo that made people shrink back in such horror? How would I know?

The good doctor, quite unaware of the undercurrent of my thoughts, went out of the way to assuage me.

"Let me tell you," he proceeded, "it's not as bad as you seem to think. Fortunately, the malignancy was localized with no visible traces of disease found elsewhere, and the lymph nodes around were free of disease, too."

He read out from the report which said:

"Well-differentiated (1) adenocarcinoma (2) – Sigmoid colon – Stage II-A (3)"

The jargon made little sense to me. I knew cancer staging ranged from I to IV, but whatever would II-A mean?

"II A is borderline between stage I and stage II," he explained. "It is stage II rather than stage I because the tumour was a little too large for stage I. It did not, however, involve the outside wall of the colon."

The gastroenterologist would not, however, take a stand on whether or not I would need chemo.

"I'm afraid, it is not my domain. The onus of the decision rests on the oncologist," he added.

He paused for a while and went on. "You should thank your stars for the timely diagnosis. Any time later would have been much worse."

I thanked the doctor for his kind words, though I could not help wondering all the same what I should thank my stars for when the biopsy report had confirmed I had cancer.

಄ ಄ ಄

The hospital had no full-fledged cancer wing at that point of time, and the lone, female oncologist was a new appointee. She walked into my room, introduced herself, and asked me if I had seen the biopsy report. She spoke an accent that sounded typically American. She had a copy of the report, and she took a good look at it.

"How about your family history? Any known cases of cancer in your family?"

I told her about my father and my sister.

"Do you have children?"

I told her how old my children were, and where they lived.

> "The first thing you should do is tell them to get screened for colon cancer, as it seems to run in the family. The sooner this is done, the better for them."

> "As for you," she went on, "it's my considered opinion that you do not need adjuvant chemotherapy. You do need to be under surveillance (4), however, until we are certain there is no more risk."

What a relief to be told I would not need chemo! I felt like getting off my bed and celebrating. If I could, I would get on to the roof of the world, and proclaim to the world at large, "Look, my cancer is gone, and I don't need chemo!"

This momentary joy came to an end, however, when I recalled, a little later, what the surgeon had said earlier. Didn't he say in no uncertain terms that I would need chemo? But who mattered more where chemo was concerned? The surgeon or the oncologist? The oncologist, of course! I was more than pleased with this young oncologist. She had freed me from the potential onslaughts of chemo.

Now, what about the surveillance the oncologist was talking about? How long would I need to be under surveillance? I turned to her for an explanation.

"In medical terminology," she said, "'surveillance' means being under continual monitoring of disease over a period of time. Where cancer is concerned, the normal period of monitoring is about five years. Initially, it would be quarterly, that is to say once every three months"

"In your case, it's going to be quarterly, that is once every three months."

As she left, I told myself that it was this young doctor that I would have to deal with, if I chose to have my follow-up at this hospital. Going by her young looks, I would not credit her with much professional experience, and I had absolutely no idea how good she was as an oncologist. "But who cares?" I told myself, "I feel very comfortable with her, and that's what is needed just now". But truth be told, one real reason why I felt comfortable with her was that she had liberated me from chemo.

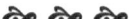

The day had more in store to make me happy. Late in the afternoon, the surgeon visited me accompanied by his assistant. He asked me if I had passed gas, and, on being told 'yes', said it was time for me to move on from liquid to solid diets. I could begin with clear fruit juice or tender coconut water, and *idlis* (steam-cooked rice cakes) for breakfast. It was also time to get off my bed and try some walking. Moving around would help prevent blood clots and enable the bowels to resume normal functions.

Between them, the surgeon and his assistant helped me sit up first and asked me to put down my feet. When, a little later, they raised me from my bed, and made me stand, I was so unsteady on my feet that I was afraid I was going to tumble and hurt myself badly. They slowly moved me out of the room to the corridor, and then up to the nurses' station about twenty yards away. When I returned to my bed after my little walk, I was immensely pleased I could walk again.

"The prognosis (5) as inferred from the pathology report is good, and the condition is treatable," the surgeon said. He consulted his assistant for a few seconds and returned to me with a broad smile.

"Well, I have some surprise for you. Your recovery is faster than expected, so you'll be discharged two days ahead, that is, the day after tomorrow."

The news sounded too good to be true. My wife, like me, was pleased. Our immediate impulse was to thank the Lord for His mercy. My prophetic wife! I recalled the loving and encouraging words she spoke to me before the treatment started. Looking back on my stay at the hospital, it had not altogether been unpleasant and, more than all, I was now 'completely cured', as the surgeon's assistant put it. I would return home in a couple of days, totally disease-free. What more would I need now? My mind was at rest, and I went to bed feeling content and grateful. That day, I slept the sleep of the innocent, and of the peaceful at heart, the first of its kind in so many days.

Chapter 4: The question of adjuvant chemotherapy

"Chemotherapy is like taking a stick and beating a dog to get rid of its fleas"-Anna Deavere Smith

Episode 1

Returning home after discharge from the hospital, I slipped back into a state of uncertainty as the question of adjuvant chemo began to loom large again. It felt nice to be told I could go without chemo, but cancer being what it is, wouldn't it be safer to take a second opinion? My family suggested it as well, and so did our doctor-neighbour who gave me a referral to an oncologist in another Coimbatore hospital. "It does not hurt to take a second or even a third opinion," my doctor-neighbour said, "and, chemo or no chemo, don't ever feel rushed to decide in a hurry." This made perfect common sense, and no sane person would ever turn a deaf ear to it. I thanked my neighbour, and I went to see the second oncologist.

The oncologist explained that even if the surgery I went through had removed all visible traces of disease, there could still be microscopic bits of cancer cells left lurking in my body. The condition might trigger further recurrences, though one could never say how soon. The main advantage of systemic adjuvant therapy, he said, was that it would minimize, if not altogether eradicate, chances of a further recurrence. He spoke at length about a 'wonder drug' (1) for colorectal cancer that had just come into use with approval from the US Food and Drug Administration (FDA) (2). It was a bit expensive, he told me, but if I could afford it, he would have it all organized for me. The costs he quoted for the drug and its administration sent my head spinning; to earn the amount I would have to continue working for my foreign employer for two more years, if not more.

The visit to the second oncologist helped confirm something beyond doubt; the chemo question carried serious implications for me, and I could ignore them only at great risk. There was however something very thorny about *why* the oncologist sounded so keen to promote a new drug while other standard drugs, much less expensive, were already available. Not that I mistrusted his intentions, but I could not help wondering whether he was trying to get me involved in a clinical trial (3) in enlightened self-interest. That apart, would the 'wonder drug' be appropriate for my condition? Clearly, what I needed now was a second opinion on the second opinion to help determine if it would be worthwhile spending a fortune on the highly touted drug.

We sought and obtained an appointment with a well-known medical oncologist in a renowned cancer care institute in Bangalore. The oncologist was a kindly soul in his late forties or early fifties. He listened to my story, viewed all paperwork including my discharge and biopsy reports, examined me physically, and asked me questions

I had never once asked myself. He confirmed the second oncologist's opinion on the need for adjuvant chemo but would not however endorse his recommendation of the wonder drug. He pointed out that the drug would not be appropriate for me as it was normally recommended for treating stage IV cancer patients. He said there were other, more appropriate options available for my condition, and they would not be as expensive.

"As regards where to have your therapy, I leave it to your choice. You can have it here or in Coimbatore," he said.

The oncologist paused for my response, but, finding none forthcoming, went on as though he had read my mind perfectly.

"Of course, it's easy for me to suggest you have the treatment here right under my care, but I know how inconvenient you may find it, as you live in Coimbatore. The right thing for you would be to have it organized in a Coimbatore hospital. About the modality of its administration, you have a choice; you may opt for chemo by IV infusion which may need hospitalization for a few hours or oral chemo which you can self-administer in the comfort of your home," he said.

Oral chemo? Self-administered in one's own place? I had not heard of such a thing before. The option would certainly suit someone like me who dreaded the very idea of visiting a hospital. I was already feeling relieved at the suggestion.

To my surprise, the oncologist volunteered to speak to the young oncologist in the hospital where I had surgery. Taking her contact number from me, he introduced himself and spoke to her. He said he agreed with her that my case was a little ambiguous but then, he said, it was his opinion that adjuvant chemo would work out to my advantage.

> "I hope," he said to her at the end, "you'll agree with me that the benefit of the doubt in matters such as this should always go to the patient".

It was amusing to hear one oncologist suggest to another that I be *poisoned* for my *benefit.* Nowhere except in medical parlance could one find poisoning suggested as a strategy to save human life. The idea sounds paradoxical, no doubt, but it assumes significance in medical science.

The oncologist hung up, and he looked satisfied with the outcome of his telephone talk. Turning to me, he said,

> "I'm glad your oncologist could take my point of view. She'll have the treatment organized for you. Meanwhile, forget all about your condition, and return to normal life. If the prognosis is any indication, everything will work out well for you. You may, if necessary, see me again after the treatment."

My visit to Bangalore put me at ease by settling the chemo question definitively. There was absolutely no chance of my saying 'no' to chemo, but, then, I had a choice as regards the modality of its administration. I could have it in a hospital or at home. I would need six cycles of chemo, to begin with, at the end of which my condition would be reviewed and more chemo would follow if the oncologist recommended it. Luckily for me, all the three oncologists I consulted were of the view that my prognosis was good, and that it would just be a matter of time for me to put my cancer behind and return to an active life.

For me, 'chemo' was yet another word as dark and mysterious as cancer. I had already known what being diagnosed with cancer was like, but about chemo, I knew next to nothing. Wanting to know more about chemo, I browsed the net, and read books for more information on the subject. There was a great deal of information on chemo: what it is and what it does, what chemo drugs are in use and how they work, what side effects chemo drugs cause and how to minimize them and so on. What however I was now most keen on knowing was information on oral chemo, particularly if it would be as effective as intravenous chemo.

What I read about oral chemo put me at ease. Though IV infusion was still the most common way of chemo administration, oral chemo was fast emerging as a more convenient option. Oral chemo might be a good option for several reasons. To begin with, it would be as good as chemo through an IV line inasmuch as it would work as efficiently. Besides, it would be relatively more hassle-free, more convenient and more timesaving, as it would involve fewer medical preliminaries and fewer hospital visits. What was more, chemo in oral form was already available for several metastatic cancers including colorectal cancer, blood cancer and breast cancer. As regards side effects, oral chemo and chemo by an IV line were not significantly different. Differences, if any, were more due to the properties of the drugs in question than to their form. Finally, oral chemo was increasingly being opted for as shown by a recent statistic. In consequence, more than one-quarter of the new drugs being studied were scheduled to come out in an oral form. Very encouraging!

Some other sources said that oral chemo might not, however, be a good option for patients taking a combination therapy (4). Such patients would anyway have to take help from a doctor, so they could on no account avoid hospital visits. Besides, the argument that oral chemo would be easier or more convenient to handle could also be faulted. This was because those opting for oral chemo would be required to take on additional responsibilities such as handling potentially complex chemo regimens and self-monitoring for potential complications. Moreover, chemo pills had to be taken at specific hours and according to specific schedules, and no chemo dose should ever be missed or increased or decreased at will. Managing side effects might also be very challenging. Not all patients or caregivers can handle such complex responsibilities.

To my mind, the advantages of oral chemo outweighed the disadvantages. For one thing, my condition did not warrant any combination chemo, so I could be treated at home. Undergoing chemo would undoubtedly be unpleasant but having it at home would be far less unpleasant than having repeated infusions in a hospital. As regards the argument that oral chemo would impose unwanted responsibility on me and my wife, the issue could be tackled by drawing a clear chemo schedule and putting it up at a place where it could not be missed. Managing side effects would not be a great issue either. In the event of the issue turning cumbersome, the oncologist could always be reached on the phone for advice.

The long and the short of my little enquiry was my eventual conviction that oral chemo would suit me better than IV infusions. I was scheduled to see my oncologist the following week, and I would consult her about it.

Chapter 5: My chemo days

"Chemotherapy is brutal. The goal is pretty much to kill everything in your body without killing you" – Rashida Jones

Episode 1

It was early April 2008 when my wife and I arrived at the hospital to see the oncologist. To get to the oncologist's office, we had to walk down a long and narrow corridor that opened into consulting rooms on either side. The passage was dimly lit and crowded far beyond its capacity with too many people moving up and down. The row of metal chairs on one side of the corridor had already been occupied, with the result that most other visitors had to laze around, obstructing the narrow passage and incommoding the passersby.

Luckily, the oncologist arrived on time, and we did not have to wait very long to see her. I was wondering how she would view my visits to other oncologists for second and third opinions, but it turned out that she had not taken it amiss. She greeted us with a warm smile and asked us to be seated.

"Of course, you have every right to seek as many opinions as you want. My opinion may differ from others', but I am still of the view that you can do without chemo. All the same, the Bangalore oncologist's opinion that you need chemo to avoid risks can't be faulted," she said.

I found her strikingly understanding, and she had a point of view I could not miss. When I hinted at my preference for oral chemo, she responded positively and came out with details of a particular chemo drug that would suit my requirements.

The drug, she said, had been successfully used in treating certain types of cancers including breast and colorectal cancers. It would attack and destroy cancer cells as well as stop them from multiplying and spreading o other parts of the body. She wrote out a prescription that said:

"Capecitabine (Xeloda) (1) – three 500 mg pills, twice a day."

"There are a few things I'd like you to know before you get started," she said.

"The pills need to be taken twice a day for two weeks in a row followed by a week's rest. The pills should be swallowed whole, maybe one by one, with plenty of water, within 30 minutes after the meal. At the end of the three weeks, the next cycle would begin."

"And about the side effects (2)," she said, "you may experience fatigue, loss of appetite, mouth ulcers, abdominal pain, constipation or diarrhoea, but their intensity may subside gradually. But do feel free to get back to me if you are too sick, or if you experience any intolerable pain or discomfort."

She reminded me again of the importance of being under surveillance during the treatment. Blood tests would have to be done at the end of each cycle. This was to gauge the way my body was responding to the treatment and to ensure that the side effects were not putting me at any grave risk.

At the end of each cycle, I should do in particular a CBC (complete blood count) test as well as liver and kidney function tests. The tests would help evaluate my overall health and detect potential disorders if any. If the results were found to be too abnormal, the treatment would have to stop for a while before further cycles started.

"Get started as early as you can," she said, "you may have to see me again after three months or even earlier if necessary. Your chemo time may really be very trying, but I'm confident you can cope with it."

At the end of the appointment, as I walked out of her consulting room, I was no longer feeling tense or anxious. For one thing, I had faith that my treatment was in safe hands and would proceed along right lines, hopefully leading to my recovery. More importantly, as I had wished, I would have my chemo cycles administered in the precincts of my house with prospects of few or no hospital visits.

Now that the battle lines had clearly been drawn between me and my cancer, I knew I was headed for a tough time, but with God, my family and my medical team joining forces with me, I was beginning to feel more and more confident that I would win the battle and emerge cancer-free at the end of the day.

ॐ ॐ ॐ

The day before my chemo sessions started, the chemo packages arrived. I opened one to see what the pills looked like. Each was a pale yellow 500 mg pill, somewhat oblong in shape. There was an information leaflet inside the package, which carried a drug description and user instructions. The drug user was instructed to keep the tablets out of the reach of children and return to the pharmacist unused tablets, if any, at the end of the treatment.

It looked like my cancer journey had put me at a crossroads. I had reached a point when I had to pause for a while and take stock of what had happened. There was now a real need to re-evaluate myself and my priorities in the light of recent developments and take appropriate decisions. The process was not just introspective, but emotional and, therefore, disturbing. What eventually emerged from the exercise was an awareness of the need to re-order my priorities in keeping with my changed circumstances.

A significant outcome of my pre-chemo introspection was my decision to quit my job abroad (3). It was a painful decision to take, but there was no way I could put it off as my chemo sessions were about to begin and might be indefinitely prolonged. Ironically, the decision was reached at a time when I needed money – lots and lots of it for my treatment and eventual recovery. Rightly, health took precedence over money which, my family said, could be found from other sources.

Closely linked to the above decision was the resolve to continue living in Coimbatore as long as needed or until the end of the treatment. Though the city was still a far cry from cities like Chennai in terms of basic hygiene, infrastructure and amenities, the place was reportedly a 'pensioners' paradise' largely in view of its temperate climate and low living costs (4). And God willing, we might even consider settling down here for the rest of our lives.

More importantly, the new circumstances afforded me a never-before opportunity to redefine family relationships and rediscover their meaning. I was increasingly becoming aware of how much I was loved. It was so reassuring to think that I was loved, not just by my family, but by others as well, including relatives and friends. It was a real family reunion as our children and their families rallied around and cheered me when I returned home after my surgery. For the first time in so many years, I could spend a great deal of quality time with people who really mattered. I realized more than ever that life was not all about pursuing a career or making money; it was much more about loving and being loved.

Most significantly, my new circumstances reawakened and deepened my spirituality. I was raised a Catholic, and my faith was a gift from my parents. Over the years, however, my spirituality had lain dormant with little or no time left for prayer, worship, meditation or devotion. Obsessed with my own worldly priorities, I had only been fleeing farther and farther from God. But no matter how evasive I had been about my spirituality, 'the Hound of Heaven' (5), relentless as He had always been, was still in hot pursuit, and it looked like I would be overrun and taken captive sooner rather than later.

Episode 2

Does it help to know what chemo is and what chemo does before actually going through it? It *does* if you ask me. What is needed is a basic idea of what going through chemo would be like, and how best one could cope with it. For me, a good deal of relevant information came from the net and my oncologist. I came to know in the first instance that the chemo experience would in most cases be devastating, not just physically but emotionally. Among other things, I would need a very strong mind to withstand the side effects which would possibly be the worst part of taking chemo. Of course, not everyone would have every side effect or would react to it in the same way. The range and intensity of the side effects might vary from patient to patient depending on their general health, age, location and stage of the disease and the type of chemo administered. Being informed helped me understand the rationale behind the treatment, learn about the potential side effects and be realistic about what to expect and how to cope with it.

It was the second week of April 2008, and I was all set to begin my first chemo cycle. I swallowed the pills readily but did not exactly know what to expect. I waited a couple of hours, but nothing much seemed to happen. I glanced through some book, switched on the TV, browsed the net, chatted with my family, played games with my grandchild and, for want of more activity, began walking up and down. It was almost lunchtime, and there was still nothing happening. Was the drug working at all (1), I wondered. It was long past my lunchtime, but I was not at all hungry. My wife kept calling me to eat, but I was least inclined to touch anything. Well, wasn't that a clear sign that I was losing my appetite? A chemo side effect? I recalled the oncologist telling me that I needed to eat regularly and stay strong, though I might not feel hungry. I had a couple of biscuits with a cup of tea and went out for a walk.

I returned home, parched and thirsty like never before, and had as much water as I could drink, until I thought I was too full. Walking does not tire me as a rule, but it was a different feeling that evening. It struck me just then. Fatigue! Another side effect? I wanted to watch the evening news, but I found that there was nothing interesting about it. I was getting more and more listless. Nothing seemed to interest me, not even interacting with my family. Could this sort of apathy be one more side effect? Now, it was eight in the evening, almost time for dinner. But the very thought of eating was nauseating (Wasn't nausea listed prominently on the list of potential side effects?). It was time for my evening dose of chemo, so I had a sandwich, a banana and a cup of milk before swallowing the pills. My children called to ask how I was doing, and I told them I was doing fine. At the end of the day, I was somewhat tired, had little or no appetite and felt a bit of nausea now and then, but it was all tolerable. I went to bed wondering if that was all about what the much-dreaded chemo could do with me.

The next morning, I got up thinking that the chemo phase might not after all be as bad as I had imagined. There was nothing remarkable about how I felt on the morning of the second day, except that I knew I was getting weaker and feeling more and more listless. I thought I had an appetite, so I had a hearty breakfast and then had my morning dose of chemo. About half an hour later, nausea reared its ugly head again, and this time around it seemed really intolerable. I was armed with antiemetic pills (2), so I thought there was no cause for alarm. Towards evening, I started experiencing a sudden mood swing – I was getting irritable for no known reason. Calls kept coming in, and answering the queries (about my condition, the treatments and their cost and the name of the hospital and the name of the specialist taking care of me) seemed so exhausting. The very sight of food was disgusting, but I had to stuff myself with something light, so I could have my evening dose of chemo before going to bed. The second chemo day was a bit different. For sure, the drug was working!

The weeks that followed turned out to be even more oppressive. Food tasted unpleasantly different, and my appetite hit rock-bottom. My mouth was sore and dry, so I was advised to use a soft toothbrush and medicated toothpaste. My weight was on the downslide as my intake of food had dwindled. My mood swings got more intensive and more frequent with the result I started isolating myself. Besides, I began to experience symptoms of a 'hand-foot syndrome' (3) which caused redness and swelling on the palms of my hands and the soles of my feet. This should have stopped my daily walk, but I went ahead despite the pain and discomfort. My sleep was yet another casualty, and I started being on sleeping pills almost every other day. However, the most annoying side effect I had was constipation which had turned chronic. I had been advised to avoid laxatives and stool softeners, so I turned to my oncologist for help. She sent me a message that said 'water, water, water' and nothing more. The meaning I construed from this cryptic message was "just keep off solid foods until the condition improved". Unfortunately, even that piece of advice did not seem to help very much.

Towards the end of my first chemo cycle, the discomfort from my constipation had turned terrible. Some visitor suggested that ripe mangoes could help ease my bowel movement. I ordered some and went ahead eating one. It was hard and unripe for the most part, and it tasted horrible. An hour or so passed before I experienced something like a bowel movement. I was happy that the mango was beginning to do the trick. However, what followed was terrifying. I began to experience what felt like a cramp, to begin with, which turned into a dreadful abdominal pain. The pain was too much to bear and I was soon left breathless. I rushed to the toilet to relieve myself, but the pain and discomfort would not stop. I staggered out of the toilet and somehow managed to get back to my bed. Now, the pain seemed to rise in a crescendo with no indication that it would subside any time soon. I was getting more and more terrified. Was it the chemo or my cancer revisiting me? I rang up my oncologist for an emergency appointment.

"You look very sick. Whatever is the matter with you?" she said.

I was too breathless to talk, so my wife explained. The oncologist listened and said she thought it was neither the chemo drug nor the cancer. Asking me to lie down, she examined me thoroughly but found no cause for alarm.

"Looks like the culprit is the carbide mango (4) you've eaten," she said.

She quickly wrote out a prescription and gave it to me.

"Calm yourself. Your pain has nothing to do with any new tumour coming up or your body reacting to the chemo. It may simply be due to food poisoning," she said.

"However," she went on, "you may have an ultrasound done if you want to. You may see me again at the end of this cycle."

The analgesic (5) I took brought me some relief. The course of antibiotics that followed helped me recover from the bout of food poisoning, and I was back to normal a few days later. How stupid of me to have swallowed one full mango artificially ripened with carbide! I vowed never to commit such indiscretions again. I went ahead and completed my first chemo cycle without any further hitch.

Looking back on it, my first chemo cycle was not that unpleasant but for the mango episode. The bottom line is that being informed may be desirable, but that is not all. There is more to feeling good and staying healthy than merely having a cartload of information on what chemo is, and what it may do. It is good to remember as well that chemo may drastically bring down your immunity levels, leaving you vulnerable to health hazards that may come from nowhere and for no known reason. It always pays to stay vigilant and circumspect and avoid circumstances that may lead to situations like the one I faced.

Episode 3

The week's rest that followed helped restore my energy in

large measure. The side effects were retreating to the background, and I was limping back to normal. It looked like my nausea had disappeared too, making way for my appetite to resurface. I was no longer that listless, and my interest in outdoor life began to re-emerge. My self-confidence which had been playing hide and seek, now ventured out into the open, almost driving me to people and places. Inexplicably, the week's rest also rekindled my interest in hobbies such as reading, writing and internet browsing which had suffered a setback for quite some time. On the physical side, I remained as feeble and fragile as before, but, strangely, that did not seem to impact on my mind negatively. I was even feeling inclined once again to indulge in strenuous activities such as long-distance walking and tidying up home. It was difficult to believe that the week's rest had elevated my morale so much, though I could not help wondering how long this phase would last.

By the end of the week, I was at the hospital again for a battery of tests. Among the labs, the most basic were the CBC and CEA tests. The former would evaluate my overall health by considering the proportions of different types of blood cells in a sample of blood. The latter would help determine how well the treatment was working for me, or if there were any indications of the cancer returning. As regards the non-lab tests, the most basic was the ultrasound scan (2) which would capture live images of the inside of my abdomen including the kidneys, liver, gall bladder, pancreas and spleen. If both types of tests showed nothing abnormal, I was told, the treatment would go on as scheduled. If, on the contrary, there were any signs of abnormality, more tests might follow, or the dosage or schedule of the cycles to come might be changed.

My first destination was the lab where I had my blood drawn for the CBC and CEA tests. Then came the ultrasound test. The sonographer (2), a man in his forties, checked my papers and asked me what my problem was. He listened to me in a matter-of-fact manner and seemed totally unmoved by my cancer story. He led me into a small, semi-dark room cluttered up with hospital equipment and a narrow, not so-clean-looking bed. Asking me to pitch on the bed, he applied some lubricating gel on my abdomen and started moving what looked like a computer mouse on the abdominal area. At the end of the procedure which hardly lasted thirty minutes, he cleaned off the gel and asked me to get up and wear my clothes. He did not appear inclined to disclose his finding as much as I did not feel like asking if there was anything sticky.

On the morning of the day I was scheduled to see my oncologist, my wife and I arrived at the hospital well in advance. The doctor was already there, and, in another half-an-hour or so, it would be my turn to see her. I glanced through the small group of cancer patients waiting to see her. What came into my view was a microcosm of the vast cancer population scattered across the length and breadth of the globe. The youngest of the group, a ten-year-old girl, had leukaemia (3), though she was blissfully unaware of the gravity of her problem. Seated just across the corridor was a young woman of about thirty-five, who had just been diagnosed with stage I breast cancer. It looked like she had not yet recovered from the shock of the diagnosis. A decrepit old man on a gurney had stage IV oral cancer, his face savagely disfigured by the disease. He had been a habitual *paan* (betel) chewer until he was diagnosed, by which time the cancer had spread to the neck and the nearby lymph nodes. Seated close to me was a fifty-year-old man who had stage III colorectal cancer. He had earlier been misdiagnosed with IBS (4) and treated for the condition for more than two years. Listening to them, I was profoundly touched by their tales of woe and impressed by their expression of hope and determination to win.

Reviewing my chemo experience, the oncologist said that the side effects I had experienced were neither unexpected nor uncommon. No doubt, my experience was unenviable, but going by my own report, it was not as bad as that of many other patients on a similar chemo plan. Unlike me, some of them could hardly eat anything and had lost considerable weight as a result. For some others, the blood counts were so erratic or so dangerously irregular that the treatment had to be interrupted for a while. As for me, she said, there was much to cheer about. My blood pressure, heart rate, body mass index, blood glucose and cholesterol levels were just normal, which was an indication that my body could tolerate the rigours of the drug.

Most significantly, I no longer had an elevated CEA, possibly because I was now in remission (5). Another pointer to this possibility was the ultrasound scan which had found nothing abnormal in my abdominal area. Of course, the CBC test results showed some lowering of the neutrophil and platelet counts, but that was pretty common in people on chemo. So, there was no need to postpone further cycles, reduce the dosage or switch to a different chemo drug. My treatment could go on uninterrupted.

> "Just push ahead despite the discomfort and inconvenience. Once the cycles are done, you'll gradually return to good health."

Buoyed up by the oncologist's words, I returned home quite determined to not let the treatment take me downhill or make me feel depressed any more. However, the side effects reappeared soon after the second cycle started, though not with as much impact as before. As I moved from cycle to cycle, I was getting weaker and weaker physically, but I told myself I would not at any cost let my body pull down my mind or depress my spirits again. Constipation continued to torment me as before and, forbidden as I was to have recourse to laxatives and stool softeners, I had to make do with home-made remedies to mitigate the problem. My mood swings started being disruptive once again, but my evening walks (6) and the relaxation techniques (7) I had picked up earlier helped me calm my nerves and rest me better. No doubt the side effects persisted throughout the cycles, but I went ahead and completed the treatment in spite of the odds. As my oncologist joked, it looked like I had become an old hand at managing chemo and its side effects.

The PET scan and other tests that followed showed that I was cancer-free. Overjoyed and unable to contain myself, I almost screamed out the question: "Doesn't that mean I'm cured?" It was an embarrassing moment for my oncologist who hastened to clarify. It was more likely, she said, I was now in remission. She explained that in medical terminology remission would mean a period of absence of symptoms of disease, a temporary recovery, but by no means a total cure. It might as well lead to an eventual cure, but one could never say anything for certain. I should be happy that I had come this far in my cancer journey.

"For any cancer patient remission is good news and so should you feel about it. The best you can do meanwhile would be to put away thoughts of the cancer, feel positive and optimistic about your future and try and live a normal life."

"I'm not sure if I can say this as a medical professional. It's not just my wish but my hunch that you've already put your cancer behind once and for all," she said, smiling.

Chapter 6: Cancer and Belief in God

"One of the main ways we move from abstract knowledge about God to a personal encounter with him as a living reality is through the furnace of affliction" - Timothy Keller: Walking with God through Pain and Suffering

Episode 1

All credit goes to our mother and our catechism (1) teachers for inculcating in me and my siblings a basic sense of religious discipline right when we were children. We were trained to wake up at the ringing of the Angeles (2), whereupon we would kneel in prayer to thank Jesus for yet another beautiful day. The diocesan church was just a stone's throw from where we lived, and we would be among the first to be there for the morning mass. Thanks to our teachers, we knew how to genuflect before the Blessed Sacrament (3), bow before the altar, and make appropriate signs and verbal responses during services. We would devoutly listen to the Biblical readings which we were expected to remember, and even repeat parts of them when called upon to do so. The mass, we were taught to believe, was the central part of the day-to-day life of Catholics, as it was a re-enactment of the sacrifice of Jesus on Mount Calvary (4). We believed, therefore, that taking part in the morning mass would strengthen us spiritually and guide us smoothly through the rest of the day while keeping us away at the same time from temptations of every kind.

Once back home from church, we would each be busy in our own way – the children getting ready for school, and our mother fixing our breakfast as well as lunch. Besides, our mother would have to get ready for her schoolwork, as she was teaching in the Catholic girls' school adjoining the church, which my three sisters attended. The Catholic boys' school where I studied was about half a kilometre from our house, and it would be a ten-minute walk for me to get there. Before breakfast, we were expected to say grace, as before every other meal of the day, the belief instilled in us being that the practice would sanctify our meal and keep our body and mind healthy. My mother and sisters would then be ready to leave for school, while I would still be taking time to finish my homework. "Won't you ever learn to do your work in time?" my mother would say very patiently. We would then pray in silence before the picture of the Sacred Heart of Jesus, pick up our satchels and, and leave together for our schools.

At my school, learning would invariably begin with a 'catechism class' taught by a cane-wielding priest who was a hard taskmaster, and whose stentorian roar would strike terror in the hearts of Catholic students. Even being late for catechism would invite the priest's wrath, who made it a point to correct such lapses by liberally using his cane.

"You should be a model to your non-Catholic schoolmates, and, woe unto you, if you misbehave," he would often say in a voice that put thunder to shame.

It was widely believed that he had put in place a vigilant espionage squad comprising senior students – mostly seminarians – whose eagle eyes would detect misbehaviour of every kind and report it to the priest promptly. How those hapless students would be dealt with was anybody's guess! Because nobody knew which of their companions would be a spy, there was mutual mistrust among friends, so everybody was well-guarded about what they did, and what they said. The result of it all was a regimented form of discipline that pervaded the entire school campus.

In the evening, we would visit the Blessed Sacrament to thank Jesus for the blessings of the day, and to reaffirm our faith in him and in the teachings of the Holy Catholic Church. We would then move on to pray at the sub-altars of saints. Each of us had our own favourite saint. Mine was Saint Antony, because I once lost a half-anna coin which I later found, *only* after praying to him. Around eight in the evening, we would sit together for a family prayer followed by hymns sung in praise of Mary, the Mother of God. I would often fall asleep during Rosary, which would annoy our mother.

> "Look," she would say more in concern than anger, "none of your sisters ever falls asleep during prayer. It's Satan, and you should resist him".

I would then rush to the bathroom to freshen up, knowing but too well that by the time I returned, the prayer would happily have ended, and it would be time for dinner. I remember asking one of our teachers once if God would be displeased with me for dozing off during prayer. Visibly amused, he said:

"Don't you worry about it my boy, for your guardian angel is there to complete the prayer for you."

I remember how I once got into serious trouble with the cane-wielding priest at school. The day the school reopened after the Easter break, news came along that the priest wanted to see me. Looking menacingly at me, the priest said,

"You were found missing for the Maundy Thursday service. Where were you that evening?"

I was dumbfounded at the question as I began to understand what the matter was all about. Well, the truth was that I had skipped church service that evening to watch a movie, but how on earth did the priest get wind of it? Finding no response forthcoming, the priest got up and advanced towards me with his formidable cane in hand. I hardly knew what was happening; my eyes blacked out suddenly, an invisible hand seemed to pull me down and I passed out in terror even before the priest got close to me. The priest called someone for help, and, between them, they carried me to a bed where I was left unconscious for a while. When I returned to my senses, the priest did not repeat his question, but gave me, to my surprise, a steaming cup of tea and biscuits. The incident brought to light the softer side of the priest that had lain concealed behind a rough exterior.

My close friend who was guilty of an equally 'heinous'
offence was not that lucky, however. An average student,
he was particularly weak in math, and his only hope after
the math test was that Jesus would work a miracle. He
carried a picture of Jesus wherever he went and prayed no
fewer than five times a day that he be spared the disgrace
of a probable failure. Man proposes, but God disposes!
When the results came out, he was in for a huge shock.
He had failed the test miserably. He wailed and lamented,
not over his misfortune, but because Jesus had let him
down! Jesus had given him a single-digit mark! I tried to
pacify him, but he would in no way be consoled. He took
out the picture of Jesus, tore it to bits and threw it into a
well on his way from school. Nobody knew how the
matter reached the priest who sent for him and flogged
him so mercilessly that the scene brought tears to my eyes.
Later, in view of the 'sacrilege' (5) committed, the priest
led my sobbing and repentant friend to the tabernacle
where we knelt and prayed in penitence.

During my transition from childhood to teenage, I would
often feel ill-at-ease whenever I went to confession (6). I
was now in junior college, almost adult-like in appearance,
voice and behaviour. The distractions of teenage came
along, and I was no longer the open, childlike, guileless boy
I once was. Every priest in the parish knew me and knew
me to be well-behaved and disciplined, so to confess my
sins to any of them would be hugely embarrassing.

Sometimes, very rarely though, I would find a visiting priest in the confessional (7), and I would seize the opportunity. Some other times, I would walk all the way down to a distant church to open up and disburden my heart of my 'ugly' sins. There were also days when I would sulk and stay away from Holy Communion because I had not confessed for quite some time. The feeling of guilt on that account began to eat into me more and more, and, unable to bear it any longer, I told my mother everything. She listened to me patiently and said:

> "It doesn't in the least matter who hears your confession. Just remember it is never a priest, but Jesus himself."

My spiritual mentor who came into my life when I was about fourteen was a young priest who was initially secretary to the bishop and later rose to the rank of a bishop and then an archbishop (8). No doubt there were other priests in the parish who helped me grow spiritually in one way or the other, but this young priest played a pivotal role in transforming me into a god-fearing, disciplined and responsible young man from a disorderly, perverse and wayward teenager. His gentle, kind and patient ways worked much better with me than intolerance, impatience and castigation. Years of tutelage under this priest also inculcated in me studiousness, diligence and perseverance which stood me in good stead and made it possible for me to sail through college creditably. His elevation as a bishop and consequent departure to the south of Tamil Nadu years later was an inexplicable personal loss leaving a void in me that never came to be filled.

The religious training I received when young helped me proceed in the right direction in search of answers to fundamental questions concerning the meaning and purpose of life. It instilled in me a fear of God, a love of fellow human beings and a sense of right and wrong. It helped me imbibe, as well, principles, values and attitudes that characterize me today as a person. That said, I need to admit that I have come a long way since the days of religious instruction under my spiritual mentor. This is no context, however, to go into details of the transformation that has come upon me except to briefly mention that it is one of my convictions now that to believe in God one does not have to be affiliated to any religion. I am still a believer, no doubt, but my faith is no longer of the kind as inherited from my mother and spiritual mentor.

Episode 2

When faced with disease and suffering, many people believe that God is there to work it out for them. Whatever their religion, their belief in God holds out an explanation for their condition; they suffer because they have displeased God in some way. These believers see disease and suffering as *punishment* from God for their sins of commission and omission. They think that just as pain is a symptom of disease, disease is but a sign of God's indignation at their sinful state. For isn't it said in the Holy Books of all major religions that sinners shall be dealt with according as they deserve? These believers hope all the same that there is no need to feel abandoned or let down, for theirs is a God who can not only cause disease but can also cure it, if he so chooses. He is not only righteous and just, but also loving and forgiving. The disease they suffer is only intended to teach them a spiritual lesson. He would forgive them if they repented of their sins and resolved never to sin again. A belief of this kind that regards disease and suffering as divine punishment and an eventual cure as a manifestation of divine forgiveness cuts across various religions including Christianity, Islam, Hinduism and Buddhism (1).

A related but by no means similar belief is that God deliberately allows or even causes sickness as a *test* of man's faith, not necessarily as punishment (2). Not only the sinner, but even the saint may be put to a test of fidelity that comes with divine sanction. The idea this time is not to castigate man for his sins, but to gauge the extent to which he is steadfast and faithful, and reward him accordingly. The suffering of Job, as recounted in the Bible, is a typical case in point. God-fearing and just, Job suffers, for no known reason, disease, humiliation, indignity and abuse. He turns to his Maker for an explanation:

> "Make me know my transgression and my sin. Why do you hide your face, and count me as your enemy?" (3).

God relents, appears before him and explains - though not in so many words - that his sickness and suffering is but a test of his faith. God is pleased with his loyalty, and Job is restored all that he once lost, including his health, and he gets much more including 'another hundred and forty years'. There are similar stories of saints and holy men being to put to test in other faiths as well.

As different from these beliefs, there is yet another that says that disease and suffering results from the *crossfire* between God and the Evil One. Man experiences pain, suffering, havoc and calamity because he lives in a world controlled by the Evil One who "walks about like a roaring lion, seeking whom he may devour" (4). And why does the Evil One do all this against man? Because he wants to alienate man from and wreak vengeance on God, his avowed, eternal enemy. In the power struggle between God and the Evil One, man gets caught in the crossfire, and hence his suffering. There is no reason for him, however, to despair, for the God he worships loves him truly and would eventually restore whatever he may have lost from the machinations of the Evil One. If only he has faith, God would intervene and rescue him from the crossfire. Isn't it said in the Holy Book that the battle only belongs to God (5)? So, the ultimate power to overrule the Evil One and protect man from suffering rests with God. This belief, too, has support from groups of all major religions.

Now, what are the implications of such popular beliefs for

cancer and cancer patients? An obvious but unacceptable implication of the *'cancer as punishment'* belief is that those who have cancer are among the worst ever transgressors of divine law. The assumption behind this belief is this: if God condemns someone to this accursed disease, they must indeed be among the most horrendous of sinners. This amounts to saying that those who do not get cancer are less sinful and better abiders of divine law. How preposterous! Just think about the case of children who get cancer, some of them at a very tender age. In what sense do they deserve it? Leave alone children, even animals get cancer, and would anyone in their right senses ever ascribe their condition to anything vicious about them? The point of it all is that anyone, good or bad, may get cancer and God has nothing whatsoever to do with it.

Equally ridiculous is the *'cancer as a test'* belief. Properly, a test should evaluate someone's worth on the basis of a set of criteria the testee is already familiar with. In the context of cancer, what are those criteria? What does the test evaluate? Is it always man's fidelity to God or anything more? And once the testee gets through the test, will he get back, as Job did, all that he once lost? There are no answers.

The case of the *crossfire* belief is the flimsiest of all. Why, in the first place, is there a struggle between God and the Evil One, and what purpose is served when man is put to suffering? And why can't the all-powerful God destroy the Evil One and put an end to man's suffering once and for all? Again, there are no answers. In brief, none of these three beliefs stands to reason when examined closely.

Beliefs of the kind as outlined above serve no purpose; at best, they can only be used as a club to beat someone with – someone you do not like or are biased against. Just a few years ago, a group of religious fundamentalists caused a storm of outrage with their allegation that the cancer of Jimmy Carter, the former US President, was indeed divine punishment for his anti-Semitism. Fortunately, the storm subsided sooner than expected because there were few takers for this insensitive and ridiculous theory. That a vast number of people across the globe eventually came together to condemn this outrage against a respected world leader is yet another story (6). Another recent example concerns Christopher Hitchens, the well-known British-American writer, whose oesophagal cancer, his enemies said, was God's punishment for his 'atheistic hate speeches'. Far from being furious, Hitchens hit back with his characteristic humour:

> "I have the cancer of the oesophagus, not larynx. Surely an omnipotent being would have better aim" (7).

Unfortunately, false religious beliefs of the kind concerning cancer are common and fanatically supported by some groups of believers, mostly religious zealots. What is fundamentally wrong with these beliefs is that they make God responsible for man's disease and suffering in one way or another. The problem is that these beliefs are, as a rule, false interpretations of religious texts, mere assumptions, very negative in approach and potentially harmful. They picture God as ruthless, vengeful, or, at least, indifferent, which typically goes against the concept of God as enshrined in the holy books of various religions. God, as religions portray, is loving, compassionate and forgiving much more than He is righteous and just.

> "Whoever does not love, does not know God, because God is love," says the Bible (1 John 4:8).

The fact remains, therefore, that God neither causes disease and suffering directly nor lets his enemy harm man in any way.

It is a different thing to say, however, that faith in God *can* help one cope with disease and suffering effectively. Among others, there are numerous cancer survivors who testify how they have benefited from their faith. Studies show, for instance, that a religious and spiritual attitude is of great help in mitigating the ravages of cancer and cancer treatments.

> "The idea of healing has never been completely medicalized. It is true that the surgeon's knife can be called healing, but even surgeons will allow that whereas cutting may be necessary for healing, it is never sufficient. This is because we are aware that healing involves our minds and our feelings – our spirits - as well as our bodies" (8).

For sure, there is more to treating and curing cancer than what surgeons and oncologists can do. Faith has a role, too, in curing disease, though one needs to be wary of what they mean by faith.

Episode 3

Studies show that faith in God has a therapeutic power that boosts immunity levels which, in turn, mitigate suffering and promote wellness (1). Psychologists say that when patients feel a sense of power outside their own lives and believe that the God they worship will answer their prayers, they begin to feel better, and they *do* get better eventually. Positive energies begin to flow through their system energizing their body, mind and spirit, and they feel strong and hopeful as never before. They get started on a journey of sustained hope and relentless effort until they reach their destination. Belief in God gets the message deeply entrenched in their subconscious mind that anything they desire is achievable as long as they are willing to make an effort, besides just believing and hoping. Joseph Murphy, a well-acknowledged spiritual psychologist (2), has this to say:

> "Give all your mental attention to recognizing the absolute sovereignty of the Spiritual Power, knowing that the God-Power has the answer and is now showing you the way. Trust it, believe in it, and walk the earth in the Light. Your prayer is already answered."

There are some believers who think that their illness is a spiritual malaise rather than a physical condition. They tend to assume on the basis of what they have read in their holy books that cure, if any, can only come from God. For isn't it written in their holy book that if someone truly believes and wishes something to happen, it will happen? (3). Some interpret the well-known saying "Doctors treat, but God heals" as meaning that what ultimately brings about healing is faith in God's power to heal, which would mean by implication that there is no need for medical intervention of any kind if one has an absolute, unassailable belief in God. They quote from their holy book that if they firmly believe and pray for something to happen, it will happen (3). They avoid hospitals and treatments like the plague until they reach a stage when they begin to feel frustrated. When, at long last, they realize their folly and decide to seek medical help, it is often very late. There are depressing stories of patients who just believed and prayed all the time with little attention paid to what needed to be done medically, and they ended up totally disappointed. Needless to say, it is risky - even dangerous - to assume that divine power is little more than magic.

It is sad but true that many cancer patients die day after day on account of their false religious beliefs. Lillian Andrews, a psychologist of repute, says:

> "Every year thousands of people die after refusing life-saving treatment on religious grounds. Even when being told 'you will die without this treatment',

patients reject the idea and believe that their God will still save them".

Is there a way to save such misguided believers from self-destruction? Andrews suggests:

"Those lives could be saved simply by classifying those people as mentally unfit for decision- making" (4).

What Andrews suggests is that these patients cannot decide for themselves as they are also mentally ill, so decisions on the medical treatment they need should be taken by someone else, preferably someone in the family.

"God helps those who help themselves," goes another familiar saying. Divine power may work by itself, but it is known to work even better alongside human effort. Here is a case study to show how divine intervention together with human effort can successfully treat and cure cancer. Felicity Corbin-Wheeler (5), the founder of *Get Well Stay Well Ministry,* was diagnosed with untreatable pancreatic cancer in 2003. Having lost her 'beautiful and very brave daughter', Melanie, to cancer in 1989, she put her trust in God and assumed responsibility for her treatment and recovery. She began to follow a nutritional therapy based on "what God tells us to eat" (6). She changed her diet to natural foods including nuts and seeds with plenty of fresh vegetable juices. Besides, she also had coffee enemas done on a regular basis and large doses of vitamin B17 and vitamin C administered from time to time.

> "Within eight months," she says, "my tumour was shrunk to a scar. A few years later I had to have a major operation to correct the damage it had done, but no trace of cancer was left in my body".

Corbin-Wheeler is still cancer-free and lives a very active life. Her book, *God's Healing Word,* bears testimony to the truth that divine power together with human effort works remarkably well.

Faith in God is healthy and desirable, but blind faith or faith based on superstitious healing practices may lead to disaster (7). No doubt, God can and does work miracles, but not in the way some faith-healers would have us believe. Studies show that the 'instant miracles' sometimes seen on television are little more than gimmicks well-choreographed and flawlessly executed on an emotional and credulous audience. There are moving reports of believers who came to great harm because they had refused medical treatment and pinned their faith not so much on God but on fake faith-healers. The American Cancer Society says:

> "Available scientific evidence does not support claims that faith healing can actually heal physical ailments. Death, disability and other unwanted outcomes have occurred when faith healing was elected instead of care for serious injuries or illnesses. When parents use faith healing in place of medical care, many

children have died that otherwise would have been expected to live. Similar results are found in adults."

For some cancer patients, "their religious belief can sometimes become a source of additional suffering", as Andrew Kneier, an eminent cancer psychologist, points out (8). Some patients, for instance, strongly believe in God's power to heal, but when the ultimate outcome does not match their expectations, they may feel frustrated. Dave, a devout Christian, had pancreatic cancer and was treated with chemotherapy. His family and friends prayed for him and Dave hoped God would listen to their prayer. But when the treatment failed, he was depressed, not so much because he was going to die, as because he thought he had been let down by God. Sarah, a believer in Judaism, had been successfully treated for breast cancer, and she was feeling grateful that God had healed her completely. But, later, when the cancer spread to her brain, and she knew she was dying, she said,

> "I'm slipping away. There is no God here. There is nothing left to do but die."

Michelle, a Buddhist, was being treated for ovarian cancer and, true to her religious tradition, she put up a brave face and endured all her suffering patiently. But when her condition deteriorated at long last, she was disappointed. "I'm a Buddhist failure," she lamented.

Now, what does research say about the impact of spirituality on treatment outcomes (9)? A study conducted at McLean Hospital in Belmont, Massachusetts, and reported in *The Journal of Affective Disorders* (2012) investigated the relationship between patients' level of belief in God and actual treatment outcomes. The subjects of the study - 159 men and women in all - were asked a single question: "To what extent do you believe in God?" One of the findings shows that "patients who had higher levels of belief in God demonstrated more effects of treatment." They were "less depressed and less likely to engage in self-harming behaviors". Equally significant was the finding that those who had faith in God also had faith in treatment. Their belief in God as well as their belief in the treatment they had helped them recover better and faster. Torrey Creed, an Assistant Professor of Psychology at the University of Pennsylvania has this to say:

> "...there's a pattern of thinking that helps people get better in treatment. And two examples of this pattern of thinking are 'I believe in treatment' and 'I believe in God'".

It is unfortunate that not all people who believe in God get cured of their ailment. There are many theological and philosophical explanations of why some people's prayers are answered, while others' are not, but they are nonetheless unconvincing. The explanation, that good people's prayers are answered, while those of the bad people are not, is not only naïve but grossly inhuman. For one thing, even the prayers of those who are known to be righteous and just may not always be heard. The Bible records two significant instances: Apostle Paul's prayer that he be cured of the 'thorn in his flesh' (10) and Saint Timothy's that he be rid of his stomach disorders (11). Neither of them was answered, and one can only wonder why.

Episode 4

Soon after I was diagnosed with cancer, anxious and well-meaning relatives and friends called to say how upsetting the news was and volunteered to help me in whatever way they could. The more religious ones came up with care and support directed towards my spiritual and emotional needs. Broadly speaking, they were of two sorts – those who had their pet theories on *why* I got cancer and others who came out with suggestions to augment my spiritual and emotional well-being. One of the first sort said that my cancer was a sign of God's love for me. Another said that it was God's effort to discipline me, and yet one more said that it was his will that I should go through this for his glory (1). From the second sort came suggestions that I pray, fast, repent, visit shrines known for miracles and take help from faith-healers. An elderly friend well-read in the Bible drew my attention to the name *Jehovah-Rapha* ('I am the Ultimate that cures you') as attributed to God in the Old Testament. Interpreting the name, he said that a real cure for any disease, let alone cancer, could come only through him and from him (2). It was gratifying to know that so many people showed an interest in adding a spiritual dimension to my cancer care.

As one believing that nothing bad ever comes from God, I never once wondered if my cancer had anything to do with my God or religion. So, none of the theories connecting my cancer with God or my *karma* as some others might put it ever bothered me. Rather than turning to religion for an explanation of why I got cancer or laying the blame on God or my *karma,* I must focus, I told myself, on what needed to be done to address the malaise. As far as I knew, there were two sides to the matter at hand - one physical and the other spiritual. As regards the physical side, I had faith that my medical team would deal with it in terms of appropriate procedures and treatments. But, not just mine, anyone's battle with cancer would have to be as much spiritual as physical. For sure, I thought, I would need a great deal of spiritual support to boost my sagging morale, elevate my low spirits and stay strong and focused no matter what happened. No doubt, part of such support would come from those who loved me, but who on earth could provide it in its entirety except God?

When I was diagnosed, I was overwhelmed by real and imagined challenges of cancer. I would often recall how my father died when still very young and go on to wonder if my life would also be interrupted before time. Not that I was scared of dying, but the uncertainty arising from the situation was getting intolerable, so I turned to God for help to clear the confusion and restore my peace. What started off as simple prayer began to assume proportions of a compulsive interaction and I became increasingly aware of a spiritual presence that constantly shadowed me - a presence that was at once reassuring and comforting. The result of it all was that all seemingly unmanageable threats began to dissipate into thin air with the further result that I emerged much stronger. Surgery seemed a threat initially, but it came and went off smoothly. The chemo phase was no doubt much harder, but the thought that the *kindly light* was there to lead me through the encircling darkness (3) and that the outstretched mighty hand (4) would unfailingly protect me from threats of all kinds helped me navigate the hard time successfully.

After a period of remission, when problems multiplied and more and more complications arose, times seemed even harder. There were moments when I was down and out, vulnerable in body and mind and desperate to the extent of questioning the very meaning of my existence. With everyone around feeling helpless, one of my friends offered to take me to a 'gifted' faith-healer, but I politely turned down his offer. I was not at all for trading my healthy belief for what I thought was morbid superstition. It is not that I discredit miracles as a rule, for I am well aware that miracles *do* happen in everyone's life - not instantly as one may wish, but naturally, over time. Looking back on my own life, I recall several instances of such an extraordinary nature, which are difficult to explain and may not have been there without the intervention of a superpower. God willing, there would be one more happening of the kind – this time restoring my health - though it was not for me to decide when or how it should happen.

I am all for prayer meetings as long as they remain dedicated to wholesome prayer. But, sadly, some of them abandon their right path and stray into the peripheries of unhealthy supernaturalism. By no means do I buy the claim that there are still people around who are endowed with powers similar to those Jesus once had. Studies show that the 'miracles' claimed by some are indeed no miracles at all. There are well-documented accounts of fake healers who fill their own coffers by capitalizing on the vulnerabilities of believers who are desperate for help. A former faith-healer explains how these pseudo-religious people trick innocent believers into ready compliance. They use the power of suggestion and hypnotic techniques to suspend their audience's critical and reasoning faculties, and then manipulate them into a "relaxed and accepting state" of mind. What eventually emerges from the process is:

> "a mindlessness that will open your audience up to suggestion...It works, so they do it and call it the Holy Spirit" (5).

It is difficult to appreciate the kind of faith that says, "I believe in God because he works miracles for me." As a matter of fact, Jesus Himself deplored such faith. He rebuked the Galileans thus:

> "Unless you people see miraculous signs and wonders...you will never believe" (6).

Another time, Jesus condemned some Pharisees using

very strong terms - "wicked and adulterous" (7) - because they would not believe unless He performed miracles in their presence. Jesus could have satisfied them easily, but he didn't, as, in his view, that was not faith. It is said that Thomas Jefferson, the third President of the US (1804-1809), compiled his own version of the New Testament by omitting sections that talk about Jesus' miracles and resurrection (8). Many wondered why Jefferson, a staunch believer, acted the way he did, but those who knew him well knew the answer. He did not want the element of supernaturalism in the holy book to overshadow and obscure its most valuable part, namely the sections that highlight the ethical system that Jesus formulated and advocated.

Incidentally, 'cancer miracles' can also happen on account of factors that have nothing much to do with religion or spirituality. There are cases of unexpected recoveries from cancer which neither religion nor medical science can explain (9). The recovery of Charles Burrows who was diagnosed with an 'inoperable liver cancer' in the summer of 2005 is a case in point. Burrows' doctors said that his cancer was untreatable and that he had just 30-60 days to live. In 2006, Burrows experienced some strange 'abdominal bloating, shaking, chills and nausea' after which his cancer disappeared miraculously.

> "I won a lottery, and I don't understand why...I would like someone to explain to me what the heck happened," a puzzled Burrows says.

In 2002, Ole Nielsen Schou was diagnosed with melanoma that had spread to his liver, abdomen, lungs, bones and brain. His doctors said that there was little more they could do. Desperate, Schou switched to complementary therapies and got started on courses of vitamins and supplements. His surprise was beyond words when it was found a few months later that about 90 per cent of his tumours had disappeared.

"It is a complete mystery. Nobody has seen anything like this," says his doctor who detailed his case in Melanoma Research (2008).

It may sound strange but it is true that some people look upon their cancer as a gift or blessing from God, says Andrew Kneier. Their reasoning is something like this: 'If God sends me cancer, there ought to be a purpose which will be revealed at an appropriate time'. What perhaps these patients mean is that there are some positive aspects to having cancer, which may not have been there except for their cancer time (10). A sixty-year-old pancreatic cancer patient once said to Kneier:

"You know, it's a shame it took cancer to hit me upside the head and show me how lucky I've been all my life."

His cancer made him look back on his life and feel grateful for the blessings he had received from God. He knew he would die soon, but his heart was full because his life had been so good. Scott Binder who was diagnosed with adenoid cystic carcinoma was equally positive about his condition which he termed his 'ultimate motivator'. Once he was diagnosed, he started living every moment of his life with 'a sense of urgency', because he knew he might not be there tomorrow.

"Having cancer is motivating me to truly embrace each moment, and I'm surprised to become as healthy as I've been," says Binder (11).

As said earlier, I no longer retain the faith I inherited from my mother and my spiritual mentor. I have now come around to believe that one's faith or spirituality can stay and flourish independently of support from or affiliation to any religion. It may not be an exaggeration to say that I owe my new outlook on spirituality and religion to my cancer time. Since I was first diagnosed, I have had plenty of time to read and reflect, which has helped reshape and refine my faith over time. Over the last few years, my spirituality has reshaped to my satisfaction, and it still keeps evolving. Significantly, this gift from my cancer has augmented my feeling of gratitude for the numerous blessings I have received from God. Like Kneier's patient, I have now acquired an equanimity that makes me accept life as it unfolds without any grumbling. Very often, though not every day, I turn to God and say:

"Thank you, Lord, for this wonderful life. I owe it all to you. My cancer is but a trifle when I recall your abundant blessings."

Chapter 7: Back into the Storm

"Part of recovery is relapse. I dust myself off and move forward again" - Steven Adler

Episode 1

Eventually, soon after my chemo cycles ended in October 2008, I began to experience unusual memory and thinking problems. It looked like my mind had turned into a lethargic and inefficient machine all on a sudden. I had difficulty, for instance, finding the right word to convey my meaning, and my verbal communication was no longer that clear or spontaneous. Strangely, even reading and writing, my all-time favourites, seemed to put me off for no reason, and the outcome from any reluctant effort made to pursue them even for a while left me disappointed. It looked like I had been transformed into an idiot, disorganized and muddled in thinking and incoherent and unclear in self-expression. My oncologist described my condition as 'chemo brain' (1), a cognitive dysfunction or mental cloudiness caused by cancer treatment, particularly chemotherapy. Those who had the condition, she said, might perceive a decrease in their mental sharpness, and some might even have difficulty remembering recent happenings. To help repair the condition, she said, I would not need medication of any kind, but activities to exercise my mind like crossword puzzles, brain games and repetitive verbal exercises could be of great help. Recalling something pleasant or interesting that happened in the past, and writing and rewriting a summary of the incident could also be helpful.

Besides, I had signs of unusual physical fatigue. The weariness was much more than what one would experience at the end of the day or after strenuous physical exercise. I found myself incapable of physical activities of the kind I had been well used to, and even the little bit of strain from my day-to-day routine would sometimes leave me exhausted. I was told it could very well be 'cancer-related fatigue' (2), a combined side effect of the cancer and the debilitating treatments that followed. It could be acute (lasting about a month) or chronic (lasting much longer). The best I could do to minimize my feeling of fatigue would be, my oncologist said, to take good care of myself - having a balanced diet, exercising moderately and relaxing whenever I could. Equally important would be the need to ensure adequate sleep by keeping my anxiety and stress levels under control. Relaxation strategies such as deep breathing, yoga or meditation might help me in this regard. Like chemo brain, cancer-related fatigue would disappear too, over time. If the recent blood test reports were any indication to go by, there was nothing much to worry about, the oncologist concluded.

Thanks to my oncologist for her sustained care and support, I was back to normal by January 2010. The quarterly test reports carried data that my body, having resumed its normal functions, was getting back to shape.

Discomfort from the chemo brain and cancer-induced fatigue began to recede too, triggering in me an urge to return to activities that had long been sidelined. Over time, my food intake and quality of sleep got better and there was an overall improvement in health. Around this time, my wife and I had moved into our own apartment flat, and our life was getting more and more organized in the new ambience. We got to know more and more people, some of whom were medical professionals who volunteered help whenever needed. With the arrival of two more grandchildren by October 2010, things were certainly looking up for us with opportunities to travel and spend time with our children and their families. I was beginning to feel so normal that I even thought of returning to my earlier job. For sure, I thought, there was no looking back as my cancer had definitely been put behind.

Around Christmas 2010, I noticed I had gained some weight. Among other things, I attributed my weight gain to the 'nutritious' foods I had been having since the treatment ended. I ate whatever I had an appetite for, including eggs, meat, fish and sugary foods, for I remembered being told by my medical team that my recovery was largely a matter of how well I ate. Before very long, my skeletal frame gradually acquired more and more substance to the extent that anyone visiting me around that time would say I was looking better. And it felt nice to be told so. I did not know at that point of time, however, that what I had been eating was a high-carb, high-fat, medium-protein and low-fibre diet which might not be the sort of nutrition that my body needed just then. I was hardly aware then of the causal relationship that cancer has with one's lifestyle, especially one's diet.

It was June 2011, about three and a half years after my diagnosis and two and a half years after my treatments had ended. I woke up at midnight when I began to experience some abdominal discomfort which later turned into a terrible pain. The pain was on and off for a while, and then it seemed to abate for a while. I closed my eyes in an effort to sleep again, but I just couldn't. I asked myself what could have caused such an unusual pain. Was it something I ate for dinner or later in the evening? It could well be so, for I remembered eating a handful of roasted peanuts just before going to bed. Roasted peanuts are hard to digest as it is, and maybe even harder to digest if consumed late in the evening, I told myself. I waited for about half an hour to see if the pain would return, but it didn't. That was a good sign, I thought, and I went back to sleep. When I got up the next morning, I was feeling normal, so there was no need to share the previous night's experience with my wife, I concluded.

The pain reappeared the next day soon after lunch. I was feeling unusually uncomfortable perhaps because I had overeaten, I thought. I took some antacids which brought on some relief, and I went back to my routine dismissing it as something insignificant. But when the pain revisited me in the middle of my sleep that night, I began to panic. I waited for it to subside, but there were more and more acute flashes of it in the next couple of hours. And the pain was getting worse as time passed. Perhaps, there was more to the nagging pain than what I ate, I thought. My wife saw me awake at that odd hour, so I had to share it all with her. She comforted me saying it might be simple indigestion, and I could see the oncologist the next day if the pain persisted. I fell back to sleep, but the pain returned after a while with such intensity that I had to go looking for some pain killer for immediate relief. We decided to seek an appointment with my oncologist as the first thing in the morning.

The next day, I called to tell my oncologist what the matter was, and she wanted a CEA test done before I saw her. The results that reached me the next day showed an elevated CEA level. I still would not believe it, so I had the test repeated at another lab and the results were more or less the same. The oncologist explained that the rise could be due to any number of reasons including inflammation or ulcers somewhere along my GI tract. She was confident that there would be nothing worrisome, but a colonoscopy would tell more, she concluded. The results of the test showed that there was nothing abnormal inside the colon, but there were indications of some abnormality on the outer wall a little above the caecum (3). After these inconclusive tests, I was finally asked to do a whole-body PET scan (4) which found

> "a *retrocaecal irregular cystic lesion with mild metabolic activity - peritoneal nodule - infected*

mucocele of appendix".

I hardly understood what the report said, but I knew for certain that there was trouble again.

Beyond doubt, there was a recurrence. Last time it was a tumour just above the sigmoid colon, but now it was some swelling or lesion on the ascending side of the colon. It looked like the vermiform appendix (5) was also cancerous. Was that an indication that the cancer had turned metastatic? From the confines of the colon, my cancer had now sneaked out, as though fed up with being a captive inside a narrow tube.

Episode 2

The news that my cancer was back started off a fresh trauma. My days of apprehensions and uncertainties returned, and it looked like I was back into the storm. What could have gone wrong? And who was to blame for this sudden reversal? Was it me, or my oncologist? Not me, certainly! I had been a compliant patient dutifully submitting myself to tests and procedures and meticulously following my medical team's advice. There was nothing more I could have done. Or was it my oncologist? The very thought was silly, as I knew she truly cared and did her very best for me. As an allopathic oncologist, she had to abide by a rigid protocol of cancer care within the limits of her system, and that was precisely what she did. Or was it God's will that I suffer again? Nothing could be more ridiculous than this because nothing bad would ever come from God. Or was it the treatments? Honestly, I did not know for sure. If these treatments had been appropriate, perhaps I would not have had a recurrence. But who was I to sit in judgement on surgery and chemo which the medical world at large viewed as standard cancer treatments? The simplest (and of course the most sensible) explanation came from one of my medical team:

"Well, you see, it is cancer, and it can only behave as cancer does" (1).

Well, it looked like I had come full circle. But where would I go from here? Back to surgery and chemo, with or without radiation? Surgery might not be as bad as chemo or radiation therapy, but there was every possibility of complications arising from anaesthesia, blood clots and infection. And whoever had emerged from an operating table totally unscathed? Of chemo, what was there to say except that it would be a real curse on cancer patients? The deadliest of the conventional cancer treatments, chemo would destroy rather than cure. I found it devastating last time, and it could be even worse this time. I had no personal brush with radiation therapy last time, so I had nothing much to say about it. All the same, I was well aware of the risks and complications that might arise from it. What a pity that cancer patients had to make do with these limited options that were neither patient-friendly nor capable of bringing forth outcomes worth all the trouble! It was depressing to think that I was back to square one after a hectic but futile cancer journey.

"It is unfortunate, but not entirely unexpected," said the oncologist with admirable frankness.

"The bitter truth is cancer cannot be prevented; it can only be treated when diagnosed," she added.

She pointed out that the cancer had now travelled outside the colon, but that was nothing much to worry about, as the condition was treatable (2). It was a matter of some comfort that the cancer was still *regional* and not *distant* (3), but its progression should be arrested before it turned metastatic. Like last time, surgery would be the first step in the treatment protocol followed by chemotherapy with or without radiation therapy, she explained.

"These unpleasant things do happen in our cancer world, and as medical professionals, we are well-used to such surprises," she said with a wry grin.

"As one who has known you for more than three years, let me tell you this is not the end of the road for you. I know you'll keep putting up a brave fight, and who knows, you may emerge a winner one fine morning," she added.

Very encouraging words indeed! But I was too engrossed in my own thoughts to pay attention to what she said. She rang up the surgeon to schedule an appointment for me.

It was a new surgeon this time, and he did not take very long to go through and grasp my medical history. Asking me to lie down, he pressed gently on the right side of my abdomen. He stopped for a while as his hand reached a point where he suspected there was something abnormal. Looking at me, he said, "Yes, I can sense it". The surgeon pointed his finger at a large area on the PET scan and told me that was where the cancer had erupted again. He drew a circle around the area on the scan, which included a part of the ileum (4), the entire caecum (5) and a length of the ascending colon.

> "I'm going to remove it all and then re-attach the remaining portion of the colon to the small intestine," he said.

The procedure (6) sounded very scary, and I wondered if the surgeon would be competent enough to cope with the challenges involved.

> "Have no fears about it. He's exceptionally skilled and has successfully handled even more complicated surgeries," said my oncologist.

I just nodded, as though the matter did not bother me that much.

My surgery was scheduled for the following week, and we started getting ready for it. We had a family council wherein everybody was convinced of the need for a second opinion on the surgery. There were a couple of questions to settle; first, if the surgery was necessary, and second, if the new surgeon could competently handle the procedure. The second opinion confirmed the need for surgery.

"You would certainly need this surgery, and the sooner this is done the better for you. Cancer being what it is, it is just a matter of time before it invades other parts of the body," the doctor explained.

The second opinion also confirmed my oncologist's personal view on the new surgeon's ability to handle the job well.

"He is very well trained as a laparoscopic surgeon, and his track record is almost impeccable," the doctor added.

The second opinion put my family at ease, though I still had doubts if everything would work out well for me.

Frankly speaking, it was really hard for me to accept the bitter truth that the cancer was back. I had heard people say that when someone's cancer was back, it was an indication that the previous treatments had failed with the cancer possibly having turned 'drug-resistant'. An obvious though unpleasant implication of such a turn of events was that the person might not survive the recurrence. Was my life drawing to a close then? And even if I survived this recurrence, there was absolutely no guarantee there would be no more recurrences. This is because, says the

American Cancer Society, we are still not certain what factors cause cancer or a cancer recurrence.

> "Even though treatment may seem to get rid of all the cancer, there may be just one tiny cancer cell left somewhere in the body. This cell might not cause any harm for many years. Suddenly, something can change the immune system and "wake up" the cell. When it becomes active, it can grow and divide to make other cells. Finally, it becomes big enough for your doctor can detect it as a recurrence" (7).

So, in effect, the cancer might reappear any time and any number of times. There was no way I could prevent it. Every time it recurred, there would be nothing much for me to do except submit myself to these 'cut, poison, burn' therapies without a murmur. My mind revolted at the very thought of these brutal, ineffective treatments. Were there any non-invasive treatment options left? None, my medical team told me. Everybody knowledgeable said the same. Anxious and tense, I browsed the net which threw up lots of information most of which seemed unscientific and therefore unreliable. Stories of cancer being cured by alternative cancer therapies were largely anecdotal, and there was no way to have them verified. For me, alternative cancer therapies were still an unchartered territory – a dark continent which I had no mind or time to explore. It looked like there was no way I could avoid these brutal conventional treatments which I totally abhorred.

Episode 3

I woke up the next morning to find myself back in my hospital room. The surgery, I was told, had been successful, though it was not laparoscopic as planned originally. At the eleventh hour, the surgeon switched plans and decided on an open surgery to avoid potential complications. Just as it happened the previous time! Personally, it wasn't good news for me. Had it been laparoscopic, it would have been much better - just a couple of days' stay in the hospital, one or two teeny wounds and less post-op pain and discomfort. But now, it looked like my hospital stay was going to be unpleasantly long as it happened last time, perhaps leading to a delayed recovery. I would once again be a captive in a hospital cell, too immobile and too powerless to be on my own. Well, there was little I could do except wait patiently until the surgeon said I could go home. I was indeed getting sick of being sick - sick of everything and everybody!

It was the same hospital as before, but the room where we were staying was located in a new block that had just come up. The view from my room was different this time; it was no longer the arterial road that throbbed with life with its unceasing traffic flows, perpetual honking of vehicles and weary pedestrians walking up and down the pavements on either side. The view now seen through the window was of the hospital parking lot which was quiet but for the noise of cars starting up and boisterous drivers breaking into sudden outbursts of laughter. The hospital had a new

'Comprehensive Cancer Care Center' set up on a fairly large area with 'facilities and equipment comparable to global standards of cancer care'. Specialist units of cancer care had now come up for radiation oncology, brachytherapy (1), medical oncology, surgical oncology and nuclear medicine (2), each staffed with specialists. The cancer care wing had a daycare facility as well, where patients received treatments until five in the afternoon. Indeed, over the last few years, the hospital had changed so much for the better.

I seemed to have changed too, though not for the better. I was no longer the positive, optimistic, intrepid person I had once been. The recurrence and the surgery had together crippled me physically and emotionally, leaving me weak in body and disoriented in mind. My outlook on life had turned so bitter and negative that I even began to distrust my medical team and their intentions. The bunch of doctors attending on me seemed unreliable, and their treatment plan a mere ploy to rob me of the little money I was left with. My mind was so full of confusion, disappointment, shock, fear, bitterness and anger that I was afraid I was going to lose my mind. It was particularly scary and unsettling to think of the treatments that would follow. I withdrew into a shell avoiding everyone. I was no longer willing to take calls, receive visitors or even talk to anyone outside the family. The only person I could confide in was my wife who kept comforting me.

"It will be well with you and your days shall be

multiplied and prolonged as the days of heaven upon the earth," she quoted from the Bible (3).

Her love and concern for me seemed the only ray of light amidst the overwhelming darkness.

I closed my eyes and fell into a reverie. I recalled the time in January 2008 when I was first diagnosed, the treatments that followed, and the subsequent three-year-long remission that brought me back to a near-normal life. It felt like I had been reborn with prospects of a new life, a life free from everything that seemed abhorrent – disease, medical procedures, treatments and hospital visits. And the new life did not last very long! It came crashing down about three and a half years later when I thought my cancer had been put behind. The diagnosis stunned me beyond words and totally upset my plans. How miserable! And now, with the second surgery done and further treatments to follow, where was I headed? The oncologist was scheduled to visit me the next day with the pathology report which might spring fresh surprises. What would my prognosis be like this time? How long would I live? And what sort of life?

The trauma specialist who visited me listened to me first before saying anything. After questioning me closely, he said the symptoms I displayed – shock, anger, anxiety, confusion, distrust and fear - were all normal reactions to the unfortunate event of an unexpected cancer recurrence.

"The problem is you assumed you'd been

permanently cured with the possibility of a recurrence never crossing your mind. When the cancer showed up again, it was such a huge shock that you just couldn't accept it."

"But this is no great cause for concern. This is very much in line with how cancer patients tend to react when there is a relapse after a period of remission. What most of them don't seem to understand is that 'remission' and 'cure' are not synonymous," he said.

Regarding my distrust of hospitals and medical professionals, he said that given my circumstances such a reaction was again normal.

"That is how most people react when they have a recurrence. The most frustrating thing about cancer is nobody including oncologists can predict a recurrence. Your doctor can only tell you what to look for by way of symptoms and get the treatment started again once they reappear. You seem to forget that your doctors are there only to help you, and you should think positively of them and their treatment methods," he said.

The trauma specialist also addressed my concern about chemotherapy.

"Yes, chemo is a mix of strong chemicals which are themselves carcinogenic (4). But the unfortunate thing is there is no viable alternative to it."

About my preference for being left alone and reluctance to talk to anyone including close friends, he said:

"It's no good keeping away from everyone. You need to talk about your feelings and concerns to at least a few you trust. Talking to someone like your friend or consulting your mental-health-care professional can help uncover the issues underlying your feelings and concerns."

The specialist gave me tips on how to reduce my trauma. He taught me the strategy of 'mindful breathing' (5) which, he said, would eliminate or minimize the unwanted thoughts that caused stress. Autosuggestion (6) which involves vocalizing positive thinking by repeating, for instance, 'God loves me', 'everybody cares for me' 'I'll be cancer-free one day' etc. would also be of immense use. Alternatively, I could spend time praying or reading the Bible. Listening to music of my choice before bedtime would also be helpful. Most importantly, I should take care to not isolate myself. He wrote out some medication which, he said, would calm my nerves and help me sleep and relax better.

"Take this drug before going to sleep, and you'll better when you get up tomorrow morning. I'll be back to see how you are doing in a couple of days," he said.

Episode 4

I got up late the next morning feeling refreshed in some measure. The first to visit me that day was the oncologist who had brought the pathology report. The report said:

well-differentiated mucinous adenocarcinoma – appendix – stage III B.

She went on to explain that 'mucinous adenocarcinoma' is a type of carcinoma made up for the most part of mucus, a greasy, gel-like secretion that forms on the lining of the inner wall of the colon. The presence of mucus was an indication that the cancer had turned aggressive, and the condition would be harder to treat than a typical carcinoma. The cancer was designated as III B because it had now grown into the outermost layer of the colon wall with potential to spread to nearby lymph nodes and other parts of the body. The appendectomy (1) done was incidental, and it would in no way affect the quality of my life.

The doctor was very positive that my condition could be treated. She was however tight-lipped about my chances of recovery. Neither was she very forthcoming about my life expectancy at this stage of colorectal cancer (2). I knew she deliberately avoided talking about it out of concern for me. Brushing aside my fears and concerns, she went on to discuss her treatment plan for me. As I feared, the discussion centred on the type of chemo best-suited for my condition.

"I know what you're thinking, but there's no way you can avoid chemo now. As your cancer has now turned invasive, you need to prevent it from spreading further, and chemo is your best option," she said.

"I wonder what benefit I would get from it when it failed me last time," I said wryly.

The oncologist looked at me as though she was not happy with what I had said.

"I understand how you're feeling, but I don't agree the chemo didn't work last time. It did, if you ask me. How then do you explain your remission of about three and a half years? If you were disease-free that long, it must have been due to strong reasons. In my opinion, the chemo you had was the principal reason."

"But, please, is there no option left?" I pleaded though I knew what she was going to say.

"No," she said emphatically. "As earlier, what you need now is a systemic therapy, and chemo would be the best for the purpose."

"I'm still not convinced," I mumbled, more in discontent than in contradiction.

"Please try to understand. I'm not forcing you into accepting chemo, but you have nothing much to choose, as a matter of fact," she said.

"Am I going back to capecitabine then?" I said.

"Not necessarily. This time you need a different chemo drug - something that's strong enough to be able to help you. I'm thinking of oxaliplatin (3) which is usually given in combination with two other anti-cancer drugs," she said.

"If it's going to be stronger than capecitabine, what about the side effects?" I said, anxious and agitated.

The oncologist seemed reluctant to provide a full account of the likely side effects. Maybe she thought a direct answer might put me off.

"I'm not directly answering your question, but as one who knows you, I'm confident you'll be able to tolerate the side effects. In any case, the side effects will get milder after the first cycle. Just in case you find the side effects intolerable at any point of the treatment, we can make suitable modifications in our treatment plan," she said.

I said I did not understand, and the oncologist hastened to explain:

"It's always possible to have the subsequent cycles put off until you recover or switch to an alternative drug."

"How will I know that the treatment is working?"

"Have no worry about it. We'll closely monitor the treatment and ascertain the results through well-coordinated tests."

"What do you think I should do to take care of myself during treatment?"

"First, you may not have a normal appetite, and food may not taste good, but you need to eat well to give yourself enough calories and enough protein, vitamins and minerals. This will help you have energy and feel active. Second, you may feel weak and uncomfortable during treatment, but take care to stay active doing whatever you like. Walking or yoga might be suitable for you to begin with. But whatever activity you choose, make sure you feel comfortable with it. And do spend time with your family and friends."

"Can I have the drug administered at home like last time?"

"I'm afraid not. Oxaliplatin does not come in pill form. It is always given by IV infusion, and you need to visit a hospital for the purpose."

Now the doctor went on to tell me about the portacath (4) which I would need for frequent and continuous chemo administration. She explained that a surgeon would implant the device in my upper chest below the collar bone in a simple surgical procedure. From the port, a catheter or tube would carry the drug to the heart through the jugular vein. The drug would then get diluted in the bloodstream and distributed to the whole body very efficiently. The portacath could also be used for blood draws and for administering antibiotics when necessary. And maintaining it would not be difficult. It only needed to be flushed every month to keep it working. She said that the port could be surgically removed when it was no longer needed.

She rang up the surgeon to schedule my portacath installation. The procedure could be done in three weeks after my discharge from hospital. Chemo infusions would start in about six weeks after my discharge from hospital. The oncologist paused for a while to see how I would react to her treatment plan. I knew what I was going to say. Here was a doctor who was very different from most other medical professionals I had seen. As a rule, doctors would go about their job in a matter-of-fact or even businesslike manner. But this doctor was not just good at her job but also very patient, caring, respectful and empathetic. I knew in my heart of hearts that what she suggested was good for me, and I accepted her treatment plan despite my deep-rooted aversion to chemo. I would give chemo another try, and, God willing, it might work this time. Or so I thought.

Chapter 8: Chemo days revisited

"What does not kill makes us stronger" - Friedrich Nietzsche

Episode 1

On a fine September day in 2011, accompanied by my wife, I checked in at the hospital for my two-day intermittent chemo infusion (1). After registration, we were shown into our hospital room and asked to wait for the oncologist to get the process started. A middle-aged nurse arrived on the scene to complete a few preliminaries. Double-checking my name, she put an ID tag round my wrist and asked me to change into a hospital gown. She asked me to read through and sign a consent form which said, among other things, that I would willingly undergo the treatment, irrespective of the consequences. She checked my blood pressure, pulse and respiration rate and went on to record my height and weight based on which the oncologist would arrive at the optimal dose of chemo my body could tolerate.

Once again, about six weeks after my previous hospitalization, I was back in a dismal hospital bed. Beside me stood the metal pole with an IV bag from which the chemo would flow into my veins uninterrupted. I had no idea what my first IV infusion was going to be like, though I knew but too well it would be anything but pleasant. Thank goodness! My hospital stay would be much shorter this time, and I would be back home in a couple of days.

The oncologist arrived sooner than expected. She greeted us warmly and bent down to examine the port nestled in my chest. Gently touching the bump on my chest, she asked me if I was feeling comfortable with the port. She numbed the skin covering the area with some gel, inserted a needle into the port and gave me my *pre-chemo* medicine (2). She said that the medicine was intended to prevent nausea and allergy-like reaction. This time around, I would receive a combination drug (2) i.e. three anticancer drugs combined into a single mix which, she said, would work better than the single drug administered earlier. Each drug had its own properties and would go about killing cancer cells in its own way. The nurse connected my port to the IV tubing, and the process started.

There you are," the oncologist said, "I don't anticipate any issues. If, however, you face any, just let me know."

About two hours into the infusion, I was feeling uncomfortable and asked the nurse to let me have a break. When the nurse unscrewed and disconnected the IV tubing, I got off my bed and went to the bathroom. When I came out, I was feeling thirsty, so I had some water and stepped out of the room for a little walk up and down the hospital corridor. When I returned to my bed about fifteen minutes later, I was feeling better, and the nurse reconnected me to the IV tubing to continue the treatment. Towards noon, the oncologist arrived back to see how I was doing. She inquired about the dosage of the drug being administered and seemed satisfied with the way the treatment was proceeding.

"It's all going on fine. I'll be back to see you in the evening before going home," she said.

True to her word, the oncologist visited me again in the evening. She asked the nurse to check my vitals and draw off blood to run a few tests to see how my body was coping. I was advised to stay hydrated meanwhile and have lots of fluids and several servings of fruits and vegetables during my stay at the hospital.

"A few small issues apart, your system seems to be responding well," she said.

It was time for the oncologist to call it a day when the nurse working the night shift appeared on the scene. The oncologist instructed her to monitor the treatment through the night, giving me short breaks as and when I needed them. After the oncologist left, my wife and I had a little chat, answered a few calls and went to bed. We were happy that the first day of my chemo infusion had passed off uneventfully.

It was after several short bouts of disrupted sleep that I got up the next morning. My eyes were gritty and swollen, and my throat parched. Nothing that I saw seemed clear, and no amount of water I gulped down my parched throat made me feel better. I had little or no appetite, so I could hardly eat anything. I was feeling not just tired, but exhausted. When the oncologist visited me a little later, she had brought with her reports of the tests ordered the previous day. The results showed some disproportion in terms of blood counts, but the matter was almost insignificant, and the treatment could go on uninterrupted, she said.

"There's nothing much to worry, as your vital signs are normal. The symptoms you're experiencing are some very common side effects which will disappear over time. Anyway, we'll have your case reviewed again tomorrow to see if there is any need to have the dosage reduced. Meanwhile, just relax and be positive. Everything will work out all right for you," she said.

I spent the rest of the day reading news magazines. One of them carried the story of an inexpensive four-herb tea that was said to cure different types of cancer. Named after the Canadian nurse, Rene Caisse, the miracle tea, *Essiac* (3), was successfully used by her to cure hundreds of terminal cancer patients. More and more cancer patients began to throng her small clinic where she treated them for little or no fee. Her meteoric rise to fame as a cancer healer roused needless jealousy and suspicion, and some local doctors brought pressure on the government to impose several restrictions on her practice. Disappointed with the way she was treated, Caisse retired from active service and went into oblivion. She died in 1978 after about 50 years of selfless service. The Canadian nurse's herbal formula eventually made its way to the US where Dr Gary Glum began to use it successfully. Like Caisse, Dr Glum had to face harassment from his Government for promoting the wonder tea. He later wrote a book, *Calling of an Angel,* narrating the story of Rene Caisse and making known the incredible healing properties of Essiac.

It was well past 8 pm, and I was still thinking of Rene Caisse and Dr Gary Glum. The saddest part of their story was that they had to face harassment from their governments for no known reason other than making a simple and inexpensive cancer remedy available. But why would anyone resist alternative therapies, if they really worked as their advocates claimed? My rumination on alternative cancer therapies ended when the nurse came in to ask if there was anything she could do before I went to sleep. I wanted to go to the bathroom, so she disconnected me and then left the room to see some other patient. As I stepped into the bathroom, I had a weird feeling that made me feel uncomfortable. I had no idea what was happening, but I could sense noisy air rushing into the cannula (4) connected to my port. Feeling dizzy and breathless, I thought I was going to collapse. My legs turned too weak to carry me, so I had to crawl back to bed. My wife was alarmed to see my condition and called the nurse for help.

When the nurse came rushing in, she at once understood

what had gone wrong. She had unknowingly left the cannula open as she disconnected me - an inadvertence that could have turned fatal (4). She apologized profusely and got in touch with my oncologist who was already in bed. It looked like the oncologist was furious to hear what had happened and alerted the duty doctor about my condition. Arriving on the scene, the duty doctor swung into action. He thumped on my chest repeatedly, turned me onto my left side, raised the head of my bed to minimize my discomfort and injected me with some drug. It seemed the oncologist had stayed awake until word reached her from the duty doctor that the first aid was successful. Before long, I fell into a deep sleep possibly because of the medication the doctor gave me. The oncologist who spoke to my wife a little later apologized for the mishap and assured her that there was no more danger. She would visit me early the next morning to see how I was doing.

When an anxious oncologist visited me the next morning, she was relieved to find me normal. She regretted the mishap the previous day, and my wife and I, on our part, thanked her for her timely action. "All's well that ends well," she said quoting from Shakespeare. When, a little later, the discussion turned on to the modality of further chemo cycles, I made it absolutely clear to her that I was no longer for an overnight stay at the hospital. She then came out with an alternative plan to suit my convenience. On day one of each cycle, I would visit the hospital daycare for chemo infusion, and, on the subsequent days, it would be oral chemo administered, as earlier, in the comfort my home. The new plan sounded better, and I accepted it.

Episode 2

The combination chemo administered between August and November 2011 was intended to destroy any microscopic cancer cells left behind after my surgery. The treatment was more intense this time, and the side effects more intolerable. The CBC tests done at the end of the first two cycles did not show any significant change in my blood counts, but the one that came at the end of the third cycle indicated, among other things, a certain deficiency of platelets (1).

> "The condition doesn't warrant breaking or postponing the treatment, but some reduction in the dosage of the chemo might be necessary," said the oncologist.

Accordingly, the dosage was brought down to suit my tolerance level, and the treatment proceeded uninterrupted.

The dosage reduction plan seemed to work well, and, by the time the fourth cycle ended, my platelet count had improved. There was no more risk, I was told, and, therefore, the earlier dosage of chemo was resumed, and I went ahead with the remaining cycles without any more disruptions. The blood work that came at the end of the treatment showed that my liver and kidney function was near-normal. However, the CBC test report indicated some *immunosuppression* (2) – a lowering of immunity.

> "The condition is a chemo-induced side effect. Now that your treatment has ended, your immunity level will likely go up again in a matter of weeks. And what is more, you're now cancer-free," said the oncologist.

It was such a relief to know I was cancer-free again and would not have to bother myself with hospital visits and medical tests and treatments until at least the end of December.

It did not take me long to understand, however, that the treatment had played havoc with my health. The drugs – oxaliplatin, in particular - had caused devastating side effects. At the end of the treatment, I was feeling so weak that, literally, even a feather could have knocked me down. I had extreme fatigue, painful mouth sores, loss of appetite, difficulty swallowing, intermittent abdominal pain and severe constipation. I could hardly eat anything, so I began to rapidly lose weight. Even small physical exertions would leave me breathless, and I was forced to rest in bed for the greater part of the day as a result.

Among the worst of the side effects was *peripheral neuropathy* (3), a condition that affects the nerves outside the brain and the spinal cord (hence, the name 'peripheral'). To begin with, it was a sensation of 'pins and needles' in my fingers and toes, and it gradually intensified and numbed my hands and feet. It would manifest itself in different ways at different times. Sometimes, it would be simple numbness, some other times, a funny tingling feeling and, yet at other times, a burning or stabbing sensation. Much worse, the condition caused a functional disorder. I had difficulty writing (The cheques I signed bounced), typing (It was no longer fast or accurate), buttoning my shirt (I needed someone's help to do this) and even walking (I had a hitherto unknown problem of balancing).

The oncologist who listened to my description of the symptoms said that I needed to wait for my overall health to get better. Meanwhile, she said, I could follow a few simple tips to ensure my functional well-being. I should keep away from sharp instruments such as knives, move around with a walking-stick, use handrails when going up or down the stairs, and watch my steps to avoid tripping. Besides, I was advised to avoid driving a car or two-wheeler until my condition got better. She suggested some oral medication to help minimize my discomfort. Just in case the condition got worse, I would need to see a neurologist, she said.

Besides, I had no normal sleep for days together. During sleep, I would sometimes bite my tongue or lower lip, and the damage done would leave me in pain or discomfort for a few days. Some other times, I would wake up with a start at any unexpected noise in the dead of night – a distant dog howling, the fan rattling over my head or even my own snoring. Or I would wake up after a terrifying nightmare – of being entangled in the thick of a battle, washed away by a raging tsunami, surrounded by weird animals or chased by deadly serpents. Strangely, one or two of the dreams kept recurring over a period of time. Not that these nightmares were in themselves scary, but, more often than not, they rendered me sleepless once I woke up from sleep.

The medical psychologist I consulted questioned me closely about any particular causes that might affect my sleep. Apart from the side effects of the cancer treatments, did I experience any pain or physical discomfort? Or was it due to any family issues that I, my wife or our children faced at the moment? Or was it on account of concern about an uncertain future or fear of imminent death? Whatever the issues, he said, I could hardly resolve any of them just by recalling them at bedtime. "What cannot be ended has to be endured," he said in a philosophical vein. To control racy thoughts disturbing my sleep and to increase my sleep time, he suggested some simple strategies.

To begin with, it would be desirable to go to bed early and make it a habit to sleep as long as possible. As a rule, it would be good to not have big meals, watch TV or work on the computer for a long time, or sleep excessively during the daytime. I could as well avoid being on the phone too long, having too much coffee, tea or other stimulants, getting into heated arguments, or watching emotionally disturbing movies or television shows. It would indeed be a great idea to set apart some time for meditation, preferably before going to bed. To prevent racy thoughts disturbing my sleep, I could, for instance, recite prayers, recall and feel grateful for God's blessings or count backwards from 100. My nightmares, he said, were just *idiopathic* (4) and would disappear on their own over time.

It was now Christmas time, an occasion to rejoice and celebrate. Three of our four children and their families had already arrived to be with us during Christmas, and we had lots of stories to exchange, both pleasant and not-so-pleasant. On Christmas Day, we attended Holy Mass, gave away Christmas gifts, played games, listened to music and stayed up late watching an evening movie on TV. The time we spent together was incredibly hilarious, and it transported me back to happy and peaceful times that had been eluding me for quite some time.

With the arrival of 2012, things appeared to be changing for the better. About three months later, I became strong enough to resume my routine. Many of the side effects had either receded or lost their intensity. The diagnostic tests, including the CEA test, indicated that my health was picking up with no visible signs of an imminent threat. Thanks to my wife and my doctors - especially my oncologist and the medical psychologist - I was no longer a mere shadow of my former self. Like the mythical phoenix, I had, once again, risen from the ashes to relive and rediscover life. I gratefully recalled the Bible verses:

> So, do not fear, for I am with you; do not be
> dismayed, for I am your God. I will strengthen you
> and help you; I will uphold you with my righteous
> right hand" (5).

Chapter 9: Into the Storm, yet again

"Courage is being scared to death...and saddling up anyway" – John
Wayne

Episode 1

How stupid of me to think that I had my cancer beaten! I
could not have been more wrong. By the end of March
2012, about seven months after my second surgery, the
CEA level in my blood was found to be rising again,
signalling an alarm. There was perhaps some error in the
measurement, I thought, so I had the test repeated at
another lab. To my surprise, the result was pretty much
the same as earlier. No need to panic or jump to any
conclusion, I told myself, as the rise could be due to any
number of causes. I waited for two more weeks and had
the test done again. Shockingly, the CEA had risen further
to a hitherto unseen level. Beyond doubt, there was
something wrong.

I wanted to see my oncologist straight away, but news
came along that she had quit her job for personal reasons.
How unfortunate! I was wondering if I could see some
other oncologist, preferably a senior doctor, and have the
issue resolved at the earliest. I was told that the hospital
had recently acquired a competent radiation oncologist,
well-qualified and well-experienced. He had previously
been with a Mumbai-based cancer centre and had just
taken over as the head of the new 'Comprehensive
Cancer Care Centre'.

The radiation oncologist suggested a PET scan (1) as the first diagnostic step. The scan report said that I had

> a *mildly hypermetabolic enlarged aortocaval node with central necrosis.*

The medical terminology was hard to decipher, so the doctor explained. The problem identified was an enlarged lymph node in the aortocaval region of my abdomen.

"A PET scan," the doctor explained, "measures metabolism, the process by which cells use sugar to produce energy. 'Hypermetabolic' implies that the cells in the area have a tendency to metabolize or use the radioactive sugar more than is normal for the particular type of cell. This would further imply that the cells in question are no longer normal".

"Central necrosis," he said, "suggests that little or no blood gets to the tissues in the central area of the infected part, possibly because the cells are dead."

"Not the entire tale the scan tells is dismal, however. The cheery part of it all is that there is no other abnormality, and the condition is still treatable," the doctor added.

"Let me also tell you this." the oncologist went on.

"The scan merely suggests some sort of cell abnormality in the area. Whether or not it is cancer can be determined only after seeing the biopsy report. The next step would be to bring in a surgeon."

When I met the surgeon a little later, he mentioned *fine-needle aspiration* (2) and laparoscopy as possible options. The former is a biopsy procedure which involves inserting a thin needle into the suspicious tissues to get a sample for evaluation under a microscope. The procedure, done under local anaesthesia, is usually considered simple and safe. The surgeon recommended the procedure, but the senior oncologist seemed to think otherwise.

> "I'd advise a laparoscopy or open surgery rather than a fine-needle aspiration. We need to have the suspicious lymph node removed first," he said.

This made sense, and, accordingly, I was scheduled for my third abdominal surgery the following week.

The pathology report which came in the wake of my surgery said:

metastatic mucinous adenocarcinoma, stage IV.

The report only confirmed the medical team's suspicion - the cancer had turned more aggressive - metastatic. As for my prognosis, the oncologist was tight-lipped. He would not tell me how many months or years I was going to live. Instead, he went on to discuss his treatment protocol for me.

> "The issue needs to be addressed without delay, and I suggest radiation (3) in the first instance. Systemic

134

treatments may follow later," he said.

Radiation therapy would be for 15-20 minutes per session for four weeks, Monday through Friday, and details of systemic treatments would be worked out later in consultation with the medical oncologist. The treatment plan sounded all right, and I accepted it. So, I was slated to begin radiation the following week. I was then taken to the treatment room for a simulation (4) which was intended to plan my treatment as well as brief me on what to expect during radiation treatment.

On the day the treatment started, I was briefed once again on the technicalities of the process and taken to the treatment room. At the centre of the room stood the linear accelerator, a huge, shiny, robot-like machine, with a long arm extended over a narrow bed-like table. A nurse helped me on to the table and, asking me to lie still, she pushed and adjusted my body until I got into the right position. I was told that just in case I felt uncomfortable about anything, I would have to raise my hand, and the radiation process would stop immediately. Once the preliminaries were completed, the radiologist and his assistants retreated into an adjoining room to get the procedure started. As the machine whirred and moved around, the outstretched arm of the machine came down to focus on my abdomen. I knew it was through this arm that radiation beams would be directed to my diseased body. In about twenty minutes, the whirring stopped, and the lights were on. I was told my first radiation session had successfully ended.

It was mid-June 2012 when the radiation treatment ended. Some of the side effects I experienced were, no doubt, distressing but on no account as intolerable as those from chemo. I was able to breeze through the first quarter of the treatment without much discomfort, but the side effects got worse as I moved on. Besides skin changes in the treated area, I also had frequent nausea, indigestion, abdominal discomfort and diarrhoea. Nothing that I was eating seemed to give me energy and strength, and the predominant feeling was one of fatigue and exhaustion. Towards the end of the treatment, I also developed a urinary problem – a tendency to urinate often and inability to regulate the flow of urine. Luckily, the problem started to subside soon after the treatment ended. Radiation also caused some permanent damage like erectile dysfunction as the nerves in the pelvic area got damaged. The oncologist explained that the treatment impacted me rather severely as it came pretty close on the heels of the surgery.

So, what next? Didn't the oncologist say, in no ambiguous terms, that I would have to follow up on the initial radiation with 'systemic treatments'? Well, I knew what he was suggesting. In cancer treatment, 'systemic treatment' is often used as a euphemism for chemotherapy. It is good patient psychology because systemic treatment' does not sound as scary as 'chemo' does. I also recalled the radiation oncologist's suggestion that I see a medical oncologist for scheduling my chemo cycles. I had gone through chemo twice already, and it was terrifying to even think of having it yet another time. Maybe it would help if I sought a second, third or even fourth opinion. Meanwhile, I would search the net for an alternative - anything I could get hold of, anything that could rescue me from the ravages of chemo. I looked and looked, but nothing seemed to offer even a ray of hope. Some inexplicable instinct kept telling me that another round of chemo might be my proverbial last straw. But who should I listen to, my doctor or my instinct? I was in a dilemma.

Episode 2

Strangely, my instinct against going through chemo yet again was getting stronger and stronger. The overall message seemed to be that I should listen to my body rather than anyone else, as the matter would not brook any more delay. Perhaps what my body was trying to tell me was that any more chemo would be disastrous, ruining my body, mind and spirit beyond repair. Was this message real, or just imagined? Would it be wise to go ahead and schedule appointments with oncologists as planned earlier, or forget all about it, and follow my own instinct? Anyway, no harm, I thought, if I listened to what other oncologists would say because the final decision on the advisability of chemo was going to be entirely mine, not theirs. If only some merciful oncologist would tell me that I could skip chemo without too much of a risk!

The oncologist I consulted first said that it would be nothing short of madness to even think of refusing chemo, as my cancer had turned metastatic. He cited the instance of someone who refused adjuvant chemo only to discover six months later that the cancer had spread to his liver. What the unfortunate patient got at that stage of disease was *palliative care* (1), and he died a few months later. The second oncologist voiced more or less the same opinion except that he offered an option - *targeted therapy* (2). Unlike standard chemo, he said, targeted therapy would target or go after and destroy *only* cancer cells. This would mean that other, healthy cells would not suffer damage, and the side effects would not, therefore, be severe. The third oncologist suggested standard chemo, targeted therapy or a combination of both. In his view, the third option would be the best ever for someone in my condition. In effect, what the three oncologists said was that there was no way I could survive without going through chemo again in one form or another.

Frustrated with unobliging oncologists beyond words, I began to explore possibilities of alternative therapies. In a country like India, where a vast majority live below the poverty line, alternative therapies which are easily accessible and relatively inexpensive are very popular. It is estimated that there are more than three million alternative therapists all over the country, practising different systems of medicine such as ayurveda, homoeopathy, naturopathy, acupuncture, diet therapy, herbal therapy, traditional Chinese medicine and so on. Other than those who are registered practitioners, there are many others who are unregistered, and they practise their own version of some system acquired from some medical professional, or from someone in the family. Most of their patients, especially those who have no access to registered medical practitioners, are drawn from the poorer sections of society. It is small wonder therefore that alternative therapies are so much in demand in India where the doctor-patient ratio is a meagre 1 to 12000 (3),

Almost all alternative therapists claim to cure cancer, though their success stories often lack credibility. Reports of successful cancer therapies appear in Indian newspapers from time to time, but they are few and far between. Besides, they are largely anecdotal - neither well-documented nor scientifically verifiable. The general opinion is that such success stories are a mere flash in the pan inasmuch as the results would not be consistent or sustainable over time. The credibility of the therapies suffers further damage with the presence of a large number of 'quacks' and 'charlatans' (4) whose knowledge of human anatomy or the system of medicine they handle is too little to result in any systematic treatment. Amidst this chaos, there is still hope that something positive may emerge from the alternative medical research initiative launched in several Indian states. In what measure and over how long a period of time the therapies being experimented with will be approved and made accessible to the common man is, however, a million-dollar question.

My search for a credible alternative cancer therapy led me to Kerala, our neighbouring state, which is regarded as a haven for alternative therapists of different kinds, both real and fake. My friend took me to someone who had a reputation of sorts as a 'healer therapist', though he had no formal qualification in medicine. He looked through my medical history and concluded, on that basis, that there was nothing much he could do to help me. What I needed at that stage of cancer was palliative care, he said. The second one said that he had successfully treated many cancer patients using his own mercury-based anticancer drug. I remembered reading somewhere that the use of metals in medicine could turn toxic leading to organ damage. The third person I met was a herbalist who claimed to have cured diseases of all kinds – including cancer – with a single herbal drug. The story sounded too amazing to be true.

Notwithstanding my initial disappointment, I went ahead with my search for some alternative therapy that had the potential to cure me. I was hoping that I would soon run into some alternative therapist who could help me recover from the ravages of conventional treatments and put me back on my road to recovery. I had been cut thrice, poisoned twice and burnt once, but with what net result? Not that these conventional treatments had been totally unhelpful, but they had indeed been too harsh, too devastating. Together they had turned my body into a toxic waste dump, crippling my mind and spirit as well. And with all this, who could say for certain that I would not have yet another recurrence? I would have none of these conventional therapies anymore, I told myself. I would change over to some alternative therapy, whatever the consequences. My instinct returned to whisper into my ear: "You've got it right at long last. It's now or never."

Chapter 10: Journey via alternative route

"Cancer is a bit like the war in Afghanistan. Attacking the tumours won't work unless you also attack the causes of the tumours. Force alone will not win the war" – Jonathan Chamberlain

Episode 1

The diagnostic tests ordered in June 2012 showed that I was cancer-free yet again. The CEA level had come down, and my kidney and liver functions were normal. Blood counts were still in disarray, but my overall health did not seem that bad. There was ground to believe that the cancer had abated, though nobody including my doctors knew how long the remission would last this time, or whether it would eventually lead to a cure. The first remission lasted about three and a half years, and the second just around seven months. The current remission could be even shorter, so there was an urgency to act - a compulsion to quit the conventional path and seek an alternative route. But what specific route would I now take - ayurveda, siddha, homoeopathy, naturopathy, acupuncture or traditional Chinese? I did not know. Whatever the choice, one thing was certain. At no point of time would I ever think of returning to conventional treatments. There was absolutely no question of any more chemo or radiation therapy for me. My family was initially against my embarking on this risky venture, but they came around to support me once I explained to them the reasons for my decision.

Meanwhile, my daughter had gathered information about a naturopath in Kerala, who had successfully treated patients with different types of cancer, using a variant of *holistic therapy* with a focus on wellness rather than illness (1)*).* An engineer by profession, he accidentally walked into alternative medicine which eventually turned out to be one of his passions. It all started with his father being diagnosed with colorectal cancer years before. His father was put through conventional treatments including surgery and chemotherapy which only pushed his body to its physiological limits. He could no longer tolerate conventional treatments, so his family had to respect his viewpoint and look for help elsewhere. Anxious to save his father's life, the young engineer started exploring different systems of traditional medicine, and eventually came out with his own version of an alternative cancer therapy. A few months into this new treatment, his father showed signs of improvement, and he was cancer-free in about a year. Encouraged by his initial success, the engineer-turned-naturopath pushed ahead and perfected his version of cancer treatment. Incidentally, his father was still cancer-free in 2012 – about 25 years after he was diagnosed.

My daughter went on to meet one of his patients, a young man of thirty-five or thereabouts who had been diagnosed with stage IV lymphoma (2), a cancer of lymph nodes. The young man had earlier been treated at a well-known Chennai hospital for more than a couple of years only to be told at the end that his condition had deteriorated.

There was nothing more the doctors could do, and he was sent home to die. It was then that he came to know about this naturopath. As the young man arrived to see the naturopath, he was on the verge of despair; he had very little hope that his life could be saved. Luckily, a few months' treatment helped him recover partially, and he returned to his job and resumed a normal life. It had been about four years since he started the new treatment, and he was still found to be cancer-free when my daughter met him.

I received all this information from my daughter without much enthusiasm. I was still harbouring doubts about the efficacy of alternative therapies, especially for life-threatening diseases such as cancer. A couple of days later, I spoke to the young man myself and emailed him a couple of times to know more of the naturopath and his methods of treatment. The reports were encouraging, but I was still undecided about meeting the naturopath and seeking his help. Time was running out, and further delay would only put me at greater risk. I came under great pressure from my family who kept telling me that I should consult the naturopath for what it was worth.

"You have nothing much to lose and possibly everything to gain if you go ahead and meet him," they said.

It was a Saturday morning, late June 2012, when I first met the naturopath at his clinic. As I entered the reception, I could not help noticing the Hippocratic dictum, 'Let food

144

be thy medicine and medicine be thy food' painted prominently on the front wall. The naturopath looked through my medical records and the sheet of paper that contained details of the treatments and the drugs I had had since I was first diagnosed in 2008. He ran a simple urine test to measure my pH level (3) which was found to be very low.

"This simple test," he said, "shows that your body is more acidic than alkaline - a condition prone to ailments of different kinds, including cancer."

"Your body is overwhelmingly toxic, largely from the treatments you've had, and, to some extent, from your lifestyle, especially your diet," he added.

He looked at me for a second and went on.

"What you need to know is that an acidic body is very conducive for cancer to grow and flourish. So, one way to keep cancer away would be to raise your pH to a neutral level (i.e. around 7.0)."

But how to raise my pH to an acceptable level?

"Detox, diet and exercise. This is the key to raising immunity and living a cancer-free life," he said.

Detoxing would mean getting rid of toxins and impurities in the body; a healthy diet with essential nutrients including vitamins and minerals would facilitate a quick recovery and regular exercise would help overcome fatigue and make one's body and mind stronger.

"To get cured, you also need to delve into its possible causes. What's now needed is a determination to change your lifestyle. And the treatment plan I'm suggesting will enable you to do it," he said.

He wrote out a long list of do's and don'ts including specifics on what I needed to drink and eat, and what to avoid.

Detox

Coffee enemas – Once a day during week 1; twice a week during week 2, 3 and 4; and once a week thereafter

(I was given a coffee enema kit, a simple device in plastic that included a bottle, a two-metre tube and a nozzle.)

2 litres of drinking water boiled with *thazhuthama* (4) leaves/ 1-2 litres of *jeera* water (water boiled with cumin seeds)/2-3 cups of green tea

3-5 glasses of mixed vegetable juice (carrots, beetroot, capsicum (peppers), apple and mint leaves/fresh lemon juice with honey

No tobacco and alcohol and no tea and coffee with milk and sugar. No processed foods including breads and pastries.

Diet

Vegan diet (without meat, fish, eggs and dairy) including a variety of fruits and vegetables, leafy greens, whole-grain products, nuts, seeds and cereals

Breakfast - 1 cup of *uppuma* (thick porridge made from broken wheat/coarse rice flour) with vegetables, especially carrot and beans)/brown rice flakes in coconut milk with 3-4 almonds/1 cup of cooked mung beans (green gram) and soymilk/orange juice/carrot/beetroot juice with ginger

Lunch - 1 - 2 cups of cooked brown rice with pepper *rasam* (pepper soup with other ingredients such as tomatoes, cumin and other spices) and steamed vegetables (preferably cruciferous vegetables (5)) and steamed greens

Dinner - 1 cup of cooked lentils/peas/chickpeas/mung beans with soy yoghurt

Fruits: bananas, papaya, guava, pineapple, berries (to be had about an hour before the main meal).

Exercise

30-45-minute walk twice a day (before breakfast and dinner)/ diaphragm breathing/meditation/yoga.

Food supplements

Medicated honey (ground cinnamon mixed in honey) - 1 tablespoonful twice a day (after breakfast and before dinner).

Grapeseed extract (300 mg) and gooseberry extract (200

mg) after breakfast; homoeopathy mineral pills (3), twice a day, preferably after breakfast and dinner

Ground turmeric (1/2 teaspoonful) mixed in honey before bedtime.

> "Far from being genetic, your problem, as I see it, is lifestyle-related. There's still time for you to change over to a healthy lifestyle. And if you do so, you may recover pretty quickly. Come back after three months to tell me how you're feeling," he said, as I took leave of him.

Although deep down I was still sceptical about the connection between lifestyle and cancer, there was something about this naturopath that made me feel I could trust him. He spoke no pompous jargon, made no tall promises and claimed no credit whatsoever for his work. There was an unmistakable air of credibility surrounding this man, his system of medicine and the way he handled his patients. Maybe his treatment plan was a godsend for me, just what I needed to put me back on my road to recovery and health. I decided to give it a go.

Episode 2

I set out on my healing journey via a naturopathic route soon after I had returned from Kerala. The journey started off well albeit not without a few initial hitches. To begin with, I was feeling a bit nervous about the coffee enema procedure (1) with the result that my first few detox tries ended up in a mess (I had to rush to the toilet even before I had taken in half the coffee solution). And getting started on a vegan diet seemed such a huge challenge. I had expected my transition to a diet sans milk, eggs, fish and meat to be smooth and hassle-free, but it turned out to be very different. Not that I envied others helping themselves with dishes of their choice, but I could not help pitying my own poor lot because what I could access when hungry was little more than half-cooked vegetables, insipid fruits or unpalatable nuts. And about the food supplements such as medicated cinnamon (2), medicated turmeric (3) and grape seed extracts (4), the less said the better. They were not just unpalatable but horribly loathsome. Most unfortunate, I even missed my morning coffee, afternoon tea and bedtime milk, as they had all been blacklisted. My taste buds, well-accustomed as they had always been to culinary delights, cried out in revolt against my decision to turn vegan.

However, it turned out that I would not need very long to get adjusted to my new regimen. Just four weeks into it, the better side of a lifestyle with a focus on detox, diet and exercise began to unfold gradually. With grit and determination, I began to follow the protocol the naturopath had suggested. I had coffee enemas, avoided acid-forming foods, exercised twice a day, practised diaphragm breathing (5), and rested well at night. Besides, I spent a good deal of time reading and, to some extent, writing. I now got active on social networking sites and even started my own blog, *Thinking Fresh,* (6) to publish some of my research papers and newspaper articles. My blogging was not so much about offering anything scholarly or even interesting to read, but much more about feeling reassured that I was well on my way to recovery. My audience, though not very large, was global, and it was gratifying to see them grow in number gradually. The only way I could explain my resurgent positivism was in terms of my new lifestyle which was beginning to impact on my body, mind and spirit significantly.

The results of the diagnostic tests ordered in September 2012 showed that I was still cancer-free. The CEA level was within the normal range, and so were the RBC and WBC counts. Surprisingly, my blood pressure and cholesterol levels were also well within the normal range - an added bonus from my new lifestyle, which I had never expected. The only hassle right now was my still abnormal platelet count - a condition that could lead to problems such as haemorrhaging and bleeding into the brain. That apart, there were a few other, though minor, glitches. I was still feeling a little weak, and my weight had dropped, though only marginally. Besides, I had experienced, from time to time, some abdominal discomfort, a feeling of being full, heavy and bloated even hours after eating – perhaps a hangover from my previous lifestyle. Perhaps my body was taking time to get adjusted to the new regimen.

It was early October 2012 when I met the naturopath

again. He ran the usual urine test which indicated a rise in my pH level. My body was no longer as acidic as earlier.

"Your system is responding well," he said, "and your gains will be even larger and more apparent in six more months."

In his view, the only real issue that needed to be fixed was my low platelet count. He suggested a simple, inexpensive home-made remedy - papaya leaf juice (7), 2-3 ounces, 2-3 times a day.

"Repeat this until your platelet count reaches 200,000," he said.

He told me that my persistent physical weakness, as well as my abdominal discomfort and bloating, would get automatically resolved in another 3-6 months. True, I had lost some weight over the last couple of months, but that was largely due to my new diet.

"Your weight may fall even further in the next few months, but that doesn't have to bother you, as long as you're feeling fit. You may see me again six months later if you really need to," he said, as I took leave of him.

My weight did indeed fall further in the following months, though my overall health was good. I was about 70 kg when I was diagnosed first in 2008, and the weight had been steadily falling since then. I weighed around 58 kg now, having lost about 2 kg since the time I took the alternative route. However, the battery of tests done in March 2013 left no room for doubt that I was still in remission, so the loss of weight might not mean anything alarming. My platelet count had dramatically risen three-fold crossing the 200,000-mark with the result that I no longer needed the papaya juice. Also, my appetite had registered an increase, and so had my energy levels. I could now walk and even jog - faster and longer. I began to haunt libraries, reading and jotting down notes for hours together. My circle of online friends and acquaintances widened, leading to a substantial increase in my networking activities. I started my second blog, *Living through Cancer: Memoirs of a Canvivor,* to share my cancer story with others. It was gratifying to see my audience growing day after day. It was such a relief to have re-found my life and re-discovered an inner peace and joy that had been eluding me for years.

The naturopath who looked over my test results said, smiling:

"Your health is as good as a young man's."

I understood that his comment, exaggerated as it might sound, was more a metaphor than a literal statement - an expression of jubilation over the remarkable change that had come upon me.

"I just couldn't have made it without your help and guidance," I said.

"You made it happen as much as I did," he said with

a modest smile.

"The secret of good health," he said, "is largely a matter of being disciplined in terms of what you think, what you eat and how you live in general. And the secret seems to have struck home with you, though rather late and at some expense."

Among other things, he suggested a few modifications in the protocol including a reduction in the intake of cinnamon and turmeric.

"Go on with your present lifestyle, and you may not need to see me again. If there's anything, call me on the phone or email me," he said.

It has been about eight years since I changed over to my new lifestyle, and I have been keeping well all the time. Of course, I have had gastrointestinal issues and other age-related problems from time to time, but never once has there been a need to see an oncologist during these years. And I have been active all the time – working out once a day, running errands or doing housework, travelling to visit our children and working on my blogs. I have had regular medical checkups and the last set of tests done a few months ago show that I am still cancer-free. I do believe that my present cancer-free condition is largely due to my changed lifestyle which has now become my way of life. I need to go on with it as it has worked for me. I will never go so far as to say that I am 'cured' but, given my understanding of the link between cancer and lifestyle, I hope to stay cancer-free as long as I live.

Summing Up

*"I've made a long voyage and been to a strange country, and I've
seen the dark man very close" - Thomas Wolfe*

As I saunter down my memory lane, I can vividly recall
the events that followed my cancer diagnosis in early
January 2008. As part of a routine medical check-up, I
was advised to go through a colonoscopy which revealed a
fairly large tumour on the descending side of my colon.
Though my doctors suspected the tumour to be
malignant, they would not say so, but I could guess what
they thought it was. The tumour was surgically removed,
and the biopsy report made it clear that it was stage IIA
colorectal cancer. I was told that what I now needed was
an adjuvant therapy – chemotherapy to be more precise –
to destroy any microscopic cancer cells left behind after
surgery. I was initially reluctant to subject myself to this
harsh procedure but accepted it eventually after my
doctors explained to me the potential risks and dangers of
skipping chemotherapy. I underwent six cycles of
chemotherapy at the end of which I was both physically
and emotionally drained. My only consolation then was
that the cancer had been driven out of my body and that I
would live disease-free thereafter.

When I was diagnosed, I was sixty-six years old, still
robust in body and mind, and teaching in a university
abroad. I had been the sole breadwinner of my family,
and with four children to raise, educate and settle in life,

my wife and I had to share hectic responsibilities and slog through a hard life. Over the years, all that we had ever wanted to do as parents had been done, and we were now looking forward to a phase of life free from oppressive responsibilities of every kind. I was waiting to quit my job abroad in a few years and return to India to settle down for a quiet life. It felt nice to think that there would be no more shuttling between countries, no more scholarly papers to write, no more gruelling deadlines to meet, no more lectures to deliver and no more teaching to do. It was at this point in my life that cancer greeted me with its ramifications looming large and threatening to interrupt my life. The cancer news made us wonder if all that we had desired and assiduously worked for would ever come about or just fade away like a dream.

A few months after the treatments, I put away all thoughts of the cancer and returned to normal life. In June 2011, after about forty months of remission, my CEA was found to be rising, and that sounded an alarm. A PET scan that followed showed that the cancer had returned. It had now crossed over to the ascending side of my colon and turned more aggressive. The earlier treatments – surgery and chemotherapy – were repeated, and I was declared cancer-free once again. But just seven months later, there was yet another recurrence which led to a third surgery to remove an infected lymph node near my spinal cord. My doctors confirmed that the cancer had turned metastatic and might spread to other parts of the body sooner rather than later. What followed was a 20-session radiation therapy which ended in June 2012. And that was not all about the treatment, I was told. As a follow-up, I would need chemotherapy and targeted therapy which together might save my life. I was stunned to hear what they said and felt betrayed by conventional therapies.

It was then that I decided to turn to an alternative. To be frank, this decision was not born of hope, but of frustration and indignation. The conventional treatments had so devastated my body, mind and spirit that I literally wanted to flee them. Flee I really wanted to, as fast and as far away as I could, but where would I go? Towards the unchartered territories of alternative medicine? I had little or no idea of any systems of alternative medicine and even less faith in their efficacy. Neither had I the time or patience to fathom their dark, weird and mazy depths to fish out a system of treatment that would suit me. When science-and- technology-based mainstream medicine had disappointed me, what help could I possibly expect from a system that was peripheral and, more importantly, not evidence-based? However, I bowed to the pressure from my family, and when, eventually, I agreed to see some alternative therapist, it was not because I was hopeful that his system would provide any relief, let alone a cure.

Contrary to what I thought, my meeting with the naturopath proved the starting point in my healing journey. The cornerstone of his system that 'food is medicine and medicine is food', and his basic philosophy that 'prevention is better than cure' appealed to me much more than any other system I had read about. The naturopath explained that what had possibly caused my condition was my lifestyle, especially my diet which had been acidic for the most part. The acidity in my body needed to be corrected so as to reactivate and augment my immunity. Amazingly, his treatment plan with its accent on *detox, diet and exercise* put me back on track within a matter of months. The good news is that about eight years into my new regimen, I am still cancer-free. Over the last few years, however, I have tinkered with and modified the original regimen to suit me better. A major deviation concerns my diet; I am no longer vegan, but pescatarian. I added fish to my diet after I sensed my body's need for more nutrition.

There is an important question, however, that I need to answer. Do I think that I am now 'cured'? My answer is "I don't know". No doubt, I have lived cancer-free for quite some time now, but it does not necessarily mean that I am cured. The simple truth is that when someone is having a remission, it does not mean that the disease has left them; it may as well be that the disease keeps lurking around for a while before it strikes again. As a matter of fact, there are numerous cancer survivors who experience a recurrence after, say, five, ten or even twenty years of remission. It is good that I remember this and keep adhering to my new lifestyle. All the same, there are moments when I feel apprehensive that the cancer may take me by surprise yet another time. Whenever something goes wrong somewhere, I begin to wonder if it is the cancer revisiting me. For me, the term, 'cancer survivor', is inadequate for it only tells a half-truth that my body is cancer-free, while it does not even hint at the state of my mind. So, I coined a special word – canvivor - (cancer survivor), a more inclusive term which, in my view, represents my state of mind and body.

My cancer journey has lasted about twelve long years now, though it has never been smooth or easy. There have been times when I stumbled and stopped midway wondering if I would ever see light at the end of the tunnel. I would have given up and succumbed to my circumstances, had it not been for the mercy of God. Every time I fell, God picked me up and put me back on my feet. In more appropriate terms, God has been supportive through people who love and care for me. First on the list is my wife who has been there for me all through the journey, nursing and nourishing me, and sharing with me my misery, pain and suffering. She has stood by me strong and solid like a rock, infusing hope and courage into me when I needed them most. 'Loving and devoted' may not adequately describe her role in my long fight against and recovery from cancer. God has also been supportive through my children and their families who have been helpful all along my cancer way. Incidentally, the idea that I publish this book for the benefit of cancer patients and survivors came from them, and, as my first readers, their suggestions have been instrumental in making this book readable.

I also need to mention my debt of gratitude to all doctors

and other medical professionals who have helped me through different stages of my journey. Though my faith in them may not always have been steady, there is no gainsaying that they have done their very best for me. I especially recall with gratitude the care and support I received from my first oncologist. She was not just my doctor, but a true friend - patient, understanding and helpful. Incidentally, we are still in touch, though she lives far away from me. Equally commendable is the role played by the naturopath who, to say the least, has helped me discover the secret of being healthy in a holistic sense. I can never forget or adequately thank him for his timely help and guidance. There are many more including relatives and friends whose greetings, wishes and prayers have contributed to my health and recovery in no small measure. I thank them all.

My journey is still on, and there may be more to tell sometime later. Meanwhile, this is my message to cancer patients and cancer survivors: 'Your cancer diagnosis is not necessarily a death sentence. There is hope for you whatever stage of cancer you may be in. Listen to your doctor by all means and listen to your body even more. Remember the decisive role that your lifestyle, especially your diet, can play in bringing about a remission or even a permanent cure. Above all, be courageous and convinced that you can beat your condition and be cancer-free as long as you live. I wish you good luck!'

Thank you for reading my cancer story.

Notes

Preface

1. Wayne Chesler's documentary, *Cut Poison Burn* gives an insider's view of the war on cancer launched in the US in the 1970s. Among other things, it throws light on the politics in the cancer *industry* that is said to have put a lid on alternative cancer treatments. You can have a glimpse of the documentary on *YouTube.*

2. 'Naturopathy' is a term variously interpreted. For me, it means a simple, active and stress-free life supplemented by a balanced vegan diet, regular exercise and good sleep.

3. Book of Job: 7: 16.

Chapter 1: Episode 1

1. Colonoscopy – Visual examination of the insides of the colon with a flexible, lighted tube inserted through the rectum. The doctor advances the tube gradually through the entire colon. The colon is inflated, so the doctor can clearly view the images of parts of the colon on the computer monitor. The procedure normally takes 30-40 minutes.

   Colonoscopy can detect colorectal cancer before it spreads to other parts of the body. It can also locate and remove polyps – small growths that can develop into cancer. A sample of the polyp is sent to the lab to determine if it is benign or malignant.

Chapter 1: Episode 2

1. Sigmoid colon – This is an S-shaped section of the colon that connects the left colon to the rectum which is the last five to six inches of the colon.

2. Sigmoidoscopy – Similar to colonoscopy, sigmoidoscopy is a visual examination of the colon using a tubular instrument called a sigmoidoscope. Unlike a colonoscopy which examines the entire colon, sigmoidoscopy examines only a part of the colon, namely the rectum and the lower colon.

Chapter 2: Episode 1

1. Colorectal cancer – This type of cancer starts in the glandular cells in the insides of the colon and/or the rectum. It usually develops from polyps that grow in the gastrointestinal tract. Polyps are usually classified into two categories: benign or non-cancerous and malignant or cancerous. Malignant polyps can develop into cancer over a period of time.

The following are some of the symptoms of the presence of colorectal cancer: i) Fatigue; ii) bloating; iii) constipation; iv) loss of appetite; v) weight loss; v) rectal bleeding.

The American Cancer Society has suggested one or more of the tests for men and women over fifty years who are not in a high-risk group: i) colonoscopy every ten years; ii) Barium enema every five years where colonoscopy is not possible; iii) Faecal occult blood test every year; iv) Sigmoidoscopy every five years.

Those in the high-risk group, that is those who have a family history of colorectal cancer, need their doctor's guidance in choosing appropriate tests.

2. Pathology report - Pathology is the study of disease with a focus on the nature, causes and development of abnormal conditions. A pathology report is written by a pathologist after examining body tissues under the microscope.

Chapter 2: Episode 2

1. Cancer types fall into three large categories; a) Carcinomas, which start in the skin and tissues that cover organs, blood vessels and glands; b) Sarcomas are cancers that affect connecting tissues including muscles and bones; c) Leukaemias and lymphomas which are cancers of the blood, bone marrow and lymph nodes.

2. 'Adenocarcinoma' is a word formed from 'adeno' meaning 'starting from a gland', and 'carcinoma' meaning cancer. It originates in glandular tissues of organs such as the lungs, colon, breast, cervix, pancreas, prostate, stomach and thyroid. It is usually diagnosed by taking a biopsy of the tumour and examining it under the microscope.

3. Adjuvant chemotherapy is formed from the two words

'adjuvant' meaning 'to aid' and 'chemotherapy'. It comes in as an additional aid after primary treatment of surgery or radiation. The idea is to minimize or destroy the microscopic cancer cells that may still lurk in parts of the body after the primary treatment.

Actor, playwright and professor Anna Deavere Smith speaks of the treatment in her show, Let Me Down Easy, thus: "Chemotherapy is like taking a stick and beating a dog to get rid of its fleas".

4. American Institute of Cancer Research (AICR) is an organization funded by the US government to aid research on the connection between diet and cancer. It takes cancer research results to the public. The gist of the organization's message is 'everyday choices can reduce our chances of getting cancer'. For more information, visit the website: www.aicr.org/

5. Complementary and Alternative Medicine (CAM) is an umbrella term for a variety of cancer treatments offered by different schools including, naturopathy, homoeopathy and Chinese herbal medicine. Details of the options and reports of their effectiveness in fighting cancer will be discussed in a separate chapter later.

Chapter 2: Episode 3

1. If cancer is diagnosed early, it can be removed with a thin, lighted tube called a laparoscope. The surgeon makes a few small cuts in the abdominal wall, through which he can view inside the abdomen, and remove the

tumour as well as nearby lymph nodes.

2. Where the disease is advanced, the surgeon may do open surgery. He makes a large cut into the abdomen to remove the tumour, and some of the healthy colon on either side. He can also check other parts of the body such as the liver to make sure the cancer has not spread.

3. The opening, called a stoma, is closed by reconnecting the healthy parts of the intestine. People who have a tumour in the lower rectum may, however, need a permanent colostomy bag which they have to carry around wherever they go.

Chapter 3: Episode 1

1. CEA – An abbreviation for carcinoembryonic antigen. CEA is a type of protein produced by cells of the gastrointestinal tract. The CEA test measures the amount of protein present in the blood of people with certain types of cancer. CEA levels may also be measured during or after cancer treatments.

2. An anaesthetist (British) or anesthesiologist (American) is a specialist who administers anaesthesia to patients who undergo surgery or a similar procedure.

Chapter 3: Episode 2

1. Catheter – A flexible tube inserted into the bladder to drain urine.

2. Dr James Esdaille (born in 1808) is considered a notable figure in the history of mesmerism. In 1830 he was appointed an assistant surgeon by the East India Company and posted in Calcutta, Bengal. He was a pioneer in the use of hypnosis for surgical anaesthesia in an era before the discovery of chloroform by James Young Simpson.

3. Chemotherapy – Chemicals administered to treat cancer. Chemotherapy works by targeting and killing rapidly dividing cancer cells. There are several different types of chemo drugs that are used in the treatment of specific types of cancer.

   Chemotherapy may be given intravenously (IV) or orally.

4. Radiation therapy – Using radiation as part of cancer treatment to control or kill cancer cells. It may be used as part of adjuvant therapy (especially after surgery) to prevent a re-occurrence of the disease. Unlike chemotherapy which is systemic (i.e. it treats the whole body), radiation therapy is localized (i.e. it treats only specific parts of the body).

5. Oncologist – A common name for a specialist in the diagnosis and treatment of cancer. A surgical oncologist is a specialist in cancer surgery. A medical oncologist specializes in the area of cancer drugs. A radiation oncologist is a specialist in radiation therapy.

Chapter 3: Episode 3

1. Well-differentiated - 'Differentiation' refers to how well the cancer cells resemble normal cells. The three degrees of differentiation are: 'poorly', 'moderately' and 'well-differentiated'. 'Poorly differentiated' means that the cancer cells in question are very chaotic and aggressive. 'Well-differentiated' cancer cells are not that aggressive and carry the best prognosis.

2. Adenocarcinoma - A common type of cancer which begins in the mucus-secreting glands in the body. Some common examples of adenocarcinoma are lung cancer, prostate cancer, oesophagal cancer and colorectal cancer. This type is known to progress rather slowly and may not show any symptoms up to about five years. Some tests that can determine colorectal cancer are colonoscopy, sigmoidoscopy and double-contrast barium enema.

3. Stage I is a small tumour confined to the inner walls of the colon, and stage IV means the disease has spread to other parts of the body. Stages II and III represent conditions between Stage I and Stage IV (See Chap 2, Episode 2 for more information).

4. Adjuvant therapy – Treatment given to the patient over a period of six to eight months usually after removing the tumour through surgery. The idea is to kill the remaining cancer cells in the body, thus lowering the risk of a recurrence. Depending upon the condition of

the patient, the oncologist may suggest chemotherapy or radiation therapy or both.

5. Surveillance – Close observation of the patient undergoing treatment. This may include a physical examination or other diagnostic tests to know the condition of the patient.

6. Prognosis – A prediction about how an illness is likely to develop and how soon it may be cured.

Chapter 4: Episode 1

1. Wonder drug – The drug, Avastin, was approved by the FDA in 2004 for treating certain metastatic cancers including colorectal cancer. It is usually given intravenously in combination with other drugs. Some of the side effects reported are increased hypertension, bowel perforation and rectal bleeding. In 2010 the FDA warned users of the drug of serious side effects including perforations in parts of the body such as the nose, stomach and bowels.

2. FDA – A federal agency of the US Department of Health and Human Services, the FDA (Food and Drug Administration) is responsible for protecting and promoting public health. It regulates facets of prescription drugs including testing, manufacturing, labelling, advertising, efficacy and safety.

3. It is a common perception that clinical trials conducted in developing countries including India are not as

transparent as in the West. The very rationale of clinical trials is that every drug should be 'evidence-based' before it is made available in the market. I remember reading reports of clinical trials being conducted in some hospitals without even taking the patients into confidence.

4. For some cancers, depending on their stage, oncologists may suggest a combination therapy i.e. combining different chemotherapy drugs into a single mix of chemotherapy and radiation therapy. The idea is to maximize the treatment effect and minimize drug resistance.

Chapter 5: Episode 1

1. Capecitabine – Otherwise known as Xeloda, the orally-administered drug is used in treating several types of cancer including colorectal, breast, gastric and oesophagal cancers. It was approved for use by the US FDA in 2005 and is on the World Health Organization's List of Essential Medicines. It works best if taken within half an hour after a meal.

2. Each person's reaction to the drug may be unique. There is a long list of potential side effects including nausea and vomiting, sore mouth and ulcers, changes in perception of taste, skin changes, loss of appetite, headaches, dizziness, weight loss, fatigue, muscle and joint pain, abdominal pain and constipation.

3. I recall how emotional I was when I decided to quit my

job. My employer was one among the best in the region, and my colleagues and students were kind, helpful and understanding. The decision marked the end of my four- decade long teaching career.

4. Having lived in Coimbatore for about eleven years now, I've come around to believe that living in this town is no longer as inexpensive as it was years ago. Some even believe that at present living in Coimbatore is more expensive than in Chennai.

5. The Hound of Heaven is a classic poem written by Francis Thompson (1859-1907). Published in 1893, the short poem speaks of how God goes after man in a never-ending pursuit, and how man keeps turning away from Him until the pursuit ends when man has to turn back to God in total surrender.

Chapter 5: Episode 2

1. If you do not experience as many side effects as some others do, you do not have to jump to the conclusion that the drug is not working. Chemo drugs have their own potential side effects, but not everyone will experience every one of them.

2. An 'antiemetic' is a drug to control nausea and vomiting. It may also be suggested to treat gastroenteritis or inflammation of the stomach and the intestines caused by a bacterial or viral infection.

3. 'Hand-foot syndrome', also called palmar-plantar

erythodysesthesia, is a side effect of certain types of chemotherapy including capecitabine. The condition causes redness, swelling and pain on the hands and/or the soles of the feet. An extreme form of the syndrome may also cause blisters.

4. According to an estimate, more than 90 per cent of mangoes coming into the Indian market are artificially ripened using a dangerous chemical called carbide. Consumption of carbide mangoes may lead to food poisoning, infection in the stomach and the intestines, diarrhoea and neurological disorders.

5. An analgesic is a pain reliever. It brings relief from pain by acting on the peripheral and central nervous systems. The doctor chooses the analgesic taking into account the nature of the pain experienced as well as the general health of the patient concerned.

Chapter 5: Episode 3

1. A CBC (complete blood count) test is intended to assess a patient's overall health and detect disorders if any. It measures a wide range of components of blood, including red blood cells, white blood cells, haemoglobin, haematocrit and platelets. It is also used in detecting cancer and monitoring cancer treatment. Chemo drugs most often result in a lowering of blood cells, triggering side effects and drastically reducing a patient's immunity.

Depending on the results, the oncologist may delay the

oncoming cycles until the condition improves.

2. A sonographer is a health professional or technician who does sonography or diagnostic ultrasound. Ultrasound uses high-frequency sound waves to look at body organs and body structure. An ultrasound test is often used in cancer treatment as a preliminary investigation to detect disorders before further tests such a CT or PET scan are ordered.

3. Leukaemia is a type of cancer that begins in the bone marrow and may lead to an abnormal rise in white blood cells which are not fully developed. Treatments of leukaemia include chemotherapy, radiation therapy, targeted therapy and bone marrow transplant.

4. IBS (irritable bowel syndrome) is a gastrointestinal disorder characterized by symptoms such as a change of bowel habits, bloating, diarrhoea, constipation and abdominal pain. What causes IBS is not well-established. However, lifestyle factors including a balanced diet, regular exercise and a stress-free life may help prevent or reduce the problem.

Because symptoms of both IBS and colorectal cancer are similar, there is every possibility of one being misdiagnosed for the other. Left untreated, IBS may lead to cancer.

5. Remission is a period in the course of a disease when it is inactive. Cancer patients are said to be in remission

when tests, physical examinations and scans show that they are cancer-free. When cancer returns after a period of remission, the condition is said to be a recurrence.

6. As a matter of fact, I should have avoided long walks while being on chemo. Because my walks were long and often strenuous, my hand-foot syndrome turned acute and very painful. At a point of time, blisters formed on both my feet and the skin peeled off leading to a suspension of my walks until a new skin formed.

7. The breathing exercise I followed was of great help in reducing stress and keeping negative feelings under control. This is done as follows: (1) The breathe-in phase during which you sit up straight and gradually inhale through your nose until the air fills your lungs; (2) The hold-phase during which you retain the air until pressure builds up and (3) The release phase during which you gradually breathe out through your nose (or mouth). You may take about 5 seconds for phase 1; 20 seconds for phase 2; and 10 seconds for phase 2. The ratio is 1:4:2. You may repeat the exercise for 5-10 minutes.

Equally beneficial is meditation which I did sitting up straight with my feet drawn close to my abdomen. What you meditate on is your choice. Most often I 'counted my blessings' (recalled the good things that happened in my life) and thanked the Lord for His abundant mercy.

The feeling that results from this is one of peace, gratitude and joy.

Besides, I listened to music, read books, reached out to family and friends on social networks, read the Bible and attended church.

Chapter 6: Episode 1

1. 'Catechism', as understood in the Catholic Church, refers to instruction on the religious doctrine of Christianity. Such instruction is usually offered through a series of questions and answers e.g. Q: Who made you; A: God; Q: What else did God make?; A: God made all things.

2. 'Angelus' is a Catholic devotional prayer at morning, noon and evening to commemorate the incarnation of Jesus. The ringing of the church bells announces the Angelus.

3. 'Blessed Sacrament' or 'Holy Sacrament' is a term used primarily in the Catholic Church. It means the Body and Blood of Christ. The Blessed Sacrament, in the form of bread, is displayed at the church altar for all Catholics to venerate.

4. 'Mount Calvary' ('Golgotha'), says the Bible, was a site outside Jerusalem where Jesus was crucified.

5. 'Sacrilege' means a violation of anything sacred or considered sacred.

6. 'Confession', as used in the Catholic Church, is the act of confessing one's sins to a confessor i.e. the priest authorized to hear confessions.

7. "Confessional' is the cubicle or place set apart inside a Catholic Church where believers make confessions to a priest.

8. Archbishop Marianus Arokiasamy (1924-2007) who became Bishop of Kottar (1970) and later Archbishop of Madurai (1987).

Chapter 6: Episode 2

1. Many Christians believe that disease is caused by man's sinful nature. Adam was the first to experience disease and suffering because he disobeyed God's command. Jesus Himself had to suffer indignity and death on account of man's sins.

Islam, again, attributes human suffering to man's disobedience to God and promises relief to those who re-submit to God and His commands (Quran, Surah 5, verse 16).

Hinduism explicates suffering on the basis of *karma* which is a moral code of cause and effect. Suffering is caused by one's own actions in this or previous lives.

Buddhism, again, attributes suffering to human desire which is a sin. The way to get over evil and suffering is by attaining nirvana. The Four Noble Truths preached by Buddhism are a diagnosis as well as a remedy for suffering.

2. All major religions subscribe to this view. The Bible, for instance, says: "God disciplines us for our good that we may share in his holiness. No discipline seems pleasant at the time, but painful. Later on, however, it produces a harvest of righteousness and peace for those who have been trained by it" (Hebrew 12: 10-11).

3. The Book of Job (1323-24).

4. 1 Peter 5-8.

5. 1 Samuel 17; 45-47.

6. https://www.youtube.com/watch?v=TJyHxm9ISvU

7. https://www.quora.com/Did-Christopher-Hitchens-get-cancer-as-a-punishment-from-God

8. Downie, R.S. (ed.) The Healing Arts; An Oxford Illustrated Anthology, p. 171. New York: Oxford University Press, 1994.

Chapter 6: Episode 3

1. "Science Proves the Healing Power of Prayer" in NewsmaxHealth, 2016. Dr Harold G. Koening, director of Duke University's Center for Spirituality, Theology and Health, says this of people who believe and pray; "In general, they cope with stress better, they experience greater well-being because they have more

hope, they are more optimistic, they experience less depression, less anxiety, and they commit suicide less often."

2. Murphy, Joseph. 2001. The Power of Your Subconscious Mind. Bantam.

3. "Truly I tell you, if anyone says to this mountain, 'Go throw yourself into the sea,' but believes that what they say will happen, it will be done for them" (Mark 11: 23).

4. "American Psychological Association To Classify Belief in God as a Mental Illness" by The News Nerd stall, July 15, 2015.

   Website: www.thenewsherd.com/health/apa-to-classify-belief-in-god-as-a-mental-illness/

5. www.felicitycorbinwheeler.org

6. Genesis 1: 29-30.

7. Taylor, Ashley. "How Faith Can Affect Therapy" in The New York Times, July 10th, 2013.

8. Kneier, Andrew. 2010. Finding Your Way Through Cancer. Berkeley: Celestial Arts.

9. www.cancerresearch.org/our-strategy-impact/people

10. Corinthians, 12: 1-6.

11. Timothy 5: 23

Chapter 6: Episode 4

1. There were a couple of others who viewed my cancer as a sign of God's wrath. A young pastor who visited me said that my condition could be due to a divine curse. "Do you believe in this kind of stuff?" I asked, more in surprise than in indignation. "Of course, I do," replied the pastor, "it's there in the Bible. Don't you believe in the Word of God?" And that shut me up. There was no way I could argue and win. Viewing what he said in retrospect, I feel that the good pastor could have avoided being so judgmental.

2. Exodus 15: 26: "The truth is that God is the one who heals. Faith is trusting the God who heals. Faith is the ultimate, absolute surrender to the God who heals. Faith is holding on to the God who can do the impossible."

3. *Lead Kindly Light* is a poem written in 1833 by John Henry Newman and turned into a hymn in 1845. When travelling in the Mediterranean, Newman fell dangerously ill and was afraid he was dying. The song strikes a note of optimism that God's unfailing power is there to guide man out of suffering and crisis. It is said that Queen Victoria wanted the poem read out to her as she was dying. It is also said to have been the last hymn sung on the Titanic before it sank.

4. Psalm: 136: 12

5. *The Word on the Word of Faith*: Ex-Faith Healer

Mark Harville Explains the Tricks of the Fake Faith Healing Trade.
www.thewordonthewordoffaithinfoblog.com/2009/05/26/ex-faith-healer.
www.deceptioninthechurch.com/sick/www.jesus-is-savior.com

6. John 4:48

7. Matthew 12: 38-39

8. Thomas Jefferson compiled "The Life and Morals of Jesus of Nazareth" (also called 'the Jefferson Bible') by cutting out sections dealing with the supernatural. In his letter to John Adams dated October 13th, 1813, Jefferson says: "In extracting the pure principles which he (Jesus) taught, we should have to strip off the artificial vestments in which they have been muffled by priests, who have travestied them into various forms, as instruments of riches and power to themselves." There are many who think that Jefferson wrote his Bible for his own satisfaction, interpreting the Christian faith as he saw it.

9. Cancer Miracles – Forbes.

www.cancerresearch.org/our-strategy-impact/people

BBC-Future-Cancer: The mysterious miracles cases.

10.Kneier, Andrew. 2010. Finding Your Way Through Cancer. Berkeley: Celestial Arts.

11. www.bbc.com/future/story/20150306-the-mystery-of-vanishing-cancer

Chapter 7: Episode 1

1. 'Chemo brain' refers to certain thinking and memory problems caused by chemotherapy. Usually, it disappears soon after the therapy ends, but may last longer in exceptional cases. Similar problems can also be caused by radiation treatment in the cerebral area.

2. 'Cancer-related fatigue' (CRF) can be experienced at any time during the treatment. It is not due to excessive physical or mental activity and not relieved by rest or sleep. Like 'chemo brain', 'cancer-related fatigue' does not usually need any medication.

3. 'Caecum' or 'cecum' is the large pouch-like area at the beginning of the large intestine.

4. 'PET' (Positron Emission Tomography) scan is an imaging test which uses a radioactive substance called a 'tracer' to look for disease in the body. The patient lies on a narrow table which slides into a tunnel-like scanner. The PET detects signals from the tracer which a computer changes into 3D pictures.

5. 'Vermiform appendix' is the three-inch tube hanging from the caecum in the lower right side of the abdomen.

Chapter 7: Episode 2

1. About whether a cancer recurrence can be prevented, the American Cancer Society has this to say: "It would be very satisfying to have something we could use to keep cancer from coming back after treatment. We want a real weapon to fight back with – something that will give us insurance against the cancer coming back. Both doctors and patients wish that there were such a magic potion or formula. But at this time, **there is nothing you could have done to make sure the cancer would not come back.** Even without current knowledge of how it develops and grows, cancer is still a mystery in many ways."

2. It is an irony that you should consider yourself lucky when your oncologist tells you that your condition is treatable. What the term 'treatable' means is that there is no immediate risk of death and that your life could be prolonged with treatments. Cancer is untreatable if it has spread widely to different locations. The treatment then assumes a new name – palliative.

3. If the cancer reappears in the original location it is called a 'local recurrence'. If it occurs in the tissues located in the vicinity of original cancer, it is said to be a 'regional recurrence'. 'Distant recurrence', as different from the other two, refers to spread (metastasis) to areas far away from the original cancer site.

4. 'Ileum' is the lowest portion of the small intestine

extending from the jejunum to the caecum.

5. 'Caecum' is the pouch-like part which begins the colon.

6. The procedure called 'right hemicolectomy' is intended to remove part of the ileum, the entire caecum and the appendix. The recovery period would be 4-6 weeks.

7. American Cancer Society.

Chapter 7: Episode 3

1. "Brachytherapy' is an advanced cancer treatment. It uses a type of energy called ionizing radiation to shrink tumours and kill cancer cells. It is used in the treatment of several types of cancer, especially prostate cancer.

2. 'Nuclear medicine' is a branch of medicine that uses small amounts of radioactive substances to diagnose and treat a variety of diseases, including many types of cancers. A radiographer carries out the scans performed in nuclear medicine.

3. Deut. 11:9, 21.

4. 'Carcinogenic' means having the potential to cause cancer. Chemotherapy and radiation therapy are carcinogenic in the sense they can trigger new tumours.

5. 'Mindful breathing' is focusing your attention on your breath while you inhale and exhale. Inhale deeply for 3 seconds, hold your breath for 2 seconds and exhale through your mouth for 4 seconds. Observe how your

chest expands and contracts.

6. Autosuggestion is a self-development strategy intended
   to create new, positive beliefs about oneself. Positive
   words and sentences are repeated again and again to
   change one's self-perception.

Chapter 7: Episode 4

1. 'Appendectomy' is the surgical removal of the
   appendix, the finger-shaped pouch that projects out
   from the caecum. The exact function of the appendix is
   not known, though it may help us recover from
   diarrhoea, inflammation and infections of the small and
   the large intestines. It is believed that the removal of the
   appendix would not impact the normal functioning of
   the human body.

2. The 5-year survival rate shows what per cent of people
   live at least 5 years after the diagnosis. The rate is about
   65% for people with colorectal cancer. The 10-year
   survival rate for them is 58%. The 5-year rate for people
   with localized colorectal cancer is 90%. If the disease
   has spread to nearby tissues or lymph nodes, the 5-year
   survival rate is 71%. If the cancer has spread to distant
   parts, the 5-year rate is 13%. The rates, however, can
   vary from patient to patient depending on other factors.

   (Source: Cancer.Net)

3. 'Oxaliplatin', a platinum-based drug, is used in the
   treatment of advanced colorectal cancer. It was

approved first in Europe in 1996 and by the US Food and Drug Administration (FDA) in 2002.

4. 'Portacath' (also called 'port') is a combination of 'port' and 'cath'. It consists of a 'portal' which has a silicone bubble for needle insertion with a 'catheter' or plastic tube attached to it. The catheter is surgically inserted into a vein, usually the jugular vein. The device makes chemo infusions convenient and efficient.

Chapter 8: Episode 1

1. When medication is intravenously administered at specific times instead of continuously over a period of time, it is said to be intermittent. The patient receiving an intermittent infusion is connected to the IV setup only when he/she is receiving an infusion. As against this, someone receiving a continuous infusion will have to remain attached to the IV setup until the infusion process is over.

2. The combination drug is called FOLFOX. It includes folinic acid (FOL), fluorouracil (F) and oxaliplatin (OX).

3. 'Essiac' (Caisse spelt backwards) is brewed from burdock root, sheep sorrel herb, elm bark and Turkish rhubarb root.

4. 'Cannula' is a metal or plastic tube inserted into the port to administer drugs or draw off blood.

5. The condition called 'embolism' occurs when an air

bubble gets trapped in a blood vessel and blocks it. Very small air bubbles can dissolve into the bloodstream harmlessly. But a large amount of air delivered into the bloodstream can lead to a life-threatening situation and may even cause death.

Chapter 8: Episode 2

1. 'Thrombocytes', otherwise known as platelets, are colourless blood cells which help form blood clots and stop bleeding. 'Thrombocytes' is a condition caused by a very low platelet count.

2. 'Immunosuppression' is a condition which results from a decrease in the ability of the bone marrow to produce an adequate number of blood cells. It may render someone vulnerable to infection and disease. It would really be a matter of concern if it happens during chemotherapy. The treatment may have to be held for a while until the condition is set right.

3. 'Peripheral neuropathy' is caused by damage to sensory nerves, motor nerves and autonomic nerves. Sensory nerves help us feel temperature, pain, vibration and touch; motor nerves help us with movement such as walking, and autonomic nerves help us perform automatic functions such as breathing.

4. An 'Idiopathic' condition arises spontaneously or is caused by an unknown factor. Diabetes, alcoholism and severe malnutrition may also cause the condition.

5. Isiah 41:10.

Chapter 9: Episode 1

1. A PET scan is a way to measure the process by which cells in the body metabolize or use sugar to produce energy. It assumes significance in cancer diagnosis because cancer cells are known to metabolize or use more sugar than healthy cells.

2. 'Fine-needle aspiration' is usually recommended to take samples of tissues in cysts, nodules or masses and enlarged lymph nodes. The sample obtained can be used to help make a diagnosis. It is relatively inexpensive and does not usually need long hospitalization.

3. 'Radiation therapy' treats cancer with high-energy waves. Most often it is administered externally with beams of radiation directed from a device called a linear accelerator to the diseased parts of the body. The energy released thus destroys cancer cells and shrinks tumours. Normal cells surrounding the affected tissues may also be affected, but they are likely to recover soon after the treatment.

   High doses of radiation also kill healthy cells as a result of which there are side effects. Not all people get all side effects.

   For more information visit www.nci.gov. Read the chapter *Radiation Therapy and You.*

4. 'Simulation' is a planning session that precedes the actual treatment. It is done to ensure that the patient

gets the best out of the treatment. Images or scans of the area to be treated are taken using a machine called a simulator. The radiation oncologist takes measurements of the area and chooses the right dose of radiation. He also makes skin markings to make sure the treatment is focused on the area. The position that the patient needs to be in during treatment is also decided during the process.

5. Isaiah 41: 10

Chapter 9: Episode 2

1. 'Palliative cancer care', also called 'comfort care' or 'supportive care', is not intended to cure or improve quality of life. It focuses on providing relief from the pain and discomfort of cancer. Though this form of care can be given at any stage of cancer, it is most often recommended for patients at advanced stages of cancer. In the West, palliative care is largely teamwork by doctors, nurses, social workers and, sometimes, spiritual people.

2. 'Targeted therapy', a special type of chemotherapy, is different from standard chemotherapy in that it is intended to destroy only the cancer cells leaving the healthy cells largely untouched. The side effects of targeted therapy may not be as severe as those from standard chemotherapy.

3. A 2012 WHO (World Health Organization) report suggested that the doctor-patient ratio should be around

1 to every 1000 people. It is said that in India there are about 939,000 registered doctors for a population of more than 1.2 billion.

4. The doctor-patient ratio is much lower in some countries – USA – 2.4:1000; Argentina – 3.8:1000; Russia - 4.3:1000.

5. Practising medicine without government approval is punishable in India under the Medical Council Act of 1954. The Indian Supreme Court ruling of 1996 condemned unauthorized medical practitioners labelling them 'quacks' and 'charlatans'.

Chapter 10: Episode 1

1. The American Cancer Society identifies five aspects of wellness: 1) physical, 2) emotional, 3) social, 4) intellectual and 5) spiritual. Physical wellness means having regular physical activity and eating well; emotional wellness is being positive about oneself and what is to come; social wellness is creating and keeping healthy relationships that facilitate a sharing of concerns, feelings, uncertainties, doubts etc.; intellectual wellness means keeping one's mind active and healthy; spiritual wellness is being aware of a greater power than one's own self and realizing it through prayer, meditation and belief in God.

2. 'Lymphoma' is a cancer that starts in cells in lymph nodes. Lymphomas are broadly of two kinds: Hodgkin lymphoma and non-Hodgkin lymphoma. Though

lymphoma can occur at any age, most cases of the disease happen to young people. It is generally treatable.

3. 'pH level' is measured on a scale ranging from 0 to 14. 7.0 is neutral. Anything above 7.0 is alkaline while anything below 7.0 is acidic. A healthy blood measuring 7.4 is more alkaline than acidic.

4. 'Thazhuthama', (Botanical name: Boerhavia diffusa), is a medicinal herb very much valued in ayurvedha. It purifies the blood and has anti-inflammatory and analgesic properties. All its parts including flowers, leaves, stem and roots have their own specific uses.

5. 'Cruciferous vegetables' are leafy green vegetables including cabbage, cauliflower, broccoli and Brussels sprouts. They are rich in nutrients such as carotenoids, vitamins C, E and K, folate and minerals. They are also a good source of fibre.

There are studies to show that cruciferous vegetables can help reduce risk in certain types of cancer including colon cancer, prostate cancer and lung cancer.

Chapter 10: Episode 2

1. In alternative therapies, coffee enemas are considered an indispensable part of cancer care protocols. Besides cleansing and healing the colon, coffee enemas are also known to eliminate parasites and detoxify and rebuild the liver.

Watch this video to know how a coffee enema is done:

https://www.youtube.com/watch?v=0OwN9ycsLgU

2. Cinnamon (cassia) mixed with honey is said to have anti-tumour, anti-diabetic, antioxidant, antimicrobial and other benefits.

   Watch this video that recommends a cinnamon compound to inhibit colorectal cancer:

   https://www.youtube.com/watchv=y8zqyIaXUMU

3. 'Turmeric' is a root crop that has been used in Indian and Chinese medicine for thousands of years. Like cinnamon, it is anti-tumour, antioxidant, and antimicrobial. There are studies to show that curcumin, the active ingredient of turmeric, is highly effective in the prevention and treatment of different types of cancer including breast, lung, liver and colon cancers.

   Watch this video:
   https://www.youtube.com/watch?v=weqqJGFz0BU

4. 'Grape seed extracts' have antioxidants that are said to prevent and cure several cancers. A team of researchers from the University of Colorado have reported in the journal, *Cancer Letters*, that grape seed extracts are effective in inhibiting colorectal cancer cells. They target the cancer cells effectively while leaving healthy cells untouched.

   Source:

5. 'Diaphragm breathing' or 'deep breathing' is done by contracting the diaphragm, a muscle located between the chest and stomach cavities. The exercise is marked by an expansion of the belly as the air enters the lungs.

   Watch this video:
   https://www.youtube.com/watch?v=kgTL5G1ibIo

6. Please visit: felixpaul41.blogspot.com

7. A normal platelet count may range from 150,000 to 450,000 platelets per microlitre of blood. An abnormally low count may lead to risks of blood clots which may eventually lead to a heart attack or stroke. Research done in 2009 at the Asian Institute of Science and Technology in Malaysia has confirmed that papaya leaf juice can increase the platelet count in patients in a short time.

   Equally good is wheatgrass juice, according to a study (2011) published in the *International Journal of Universal Pharmacy and Life Sciences.*

   Gooseberries, also known as *amla,* are also found to be of use in raising the platelet count.